MIA WILSON

THE COMPLETE KETOGENIC DIET COOKBOOK

Your Essential Keto Guide with Easy and

Budget-Friendly Recipes for Weight

Loss and Body Health

Disclaimer notice:

Please respect that the information contained within this document is for educational and enchainment purposes only. Every attempt has been made 10 provide accurate, up to date and reliable, complete information. No warranties of any kind are expressed or implied. Readers acknowledge that the author is not engaging in the rendering of legal, financial, medical or professional advice.

By reading this document, the reader agrees that under no circumstances are we responsible for any losses, direct or indirect, which are incurred as a result of the use of information contained in this document, including but not limited to errors, omissions, or any inaccuracies.

Table of Contents

INTRODUCTION..9

CHAPTER 2: KETOGENIC DIET, ETYMOLOGY....11

CHAPTER 3: BACKGROUND AND HISTORY OF THE KETOGENIC DIET 14

CHAPTER 4: BENEFITS OF ADOPTING A KETOGENIC DIET 17

CHAPTER 5: WHAT TO EAT AND WHAT NOT TO EAT ON A KETOGENIC DIET................................ 20

What you can eat on a Ketogenic diet.................. 21

What not to eat on Foods to avoid 22

Note 23

CHAPTER 6: KETOGENIC DIET BREAKFAST RECIPES...24

Recipe 1: Chocolate Chia Pudding.......................24

Recipe 2: Sweet potato Muffins...........................25

Recipe 3: Granola Bars..27

Recipe 4: Mushroom Quiche 28

Recipe 5: Almond Flour Pancakes 30

Recipe 6: Cashew Pudding....................................32

Recipe 7: Breakfast Omelette 34

Recipe 8: Gluten Free Bread 35

Recipe 9: Egg Roll 37

Recipe 10: Sweet Potato Waffles 39

CHAPTER 7: KETOGENIC DIET APPETIZERS 41

Recipe 11: Cauliflower Muffins 41

Recipe 12: Stuffed Sardines 43

Recipe 13: Spring Roll Bowl 45

Recipe 14: Stuffed Mushrooms 47

Recipe 15: Roasted Cauliflower 49

Recipe 16: Stuffed Peppers 51

Recipe 17: Roasted Squash 53

Recipe 18: Chicken Fingers 55

Recipe 19: Zucchini Fritters 57

Recipe 20: Cashew Hummus 59

CHAPTER 8: KETOGENIC DIET LUNCH RECIPES
.... 61

Recipe 21: Cauliflower Pizza 61

Recipe 22: Chicken Kabobs with Chimichurri
Sauce 63

Recipe 23: Chicken with Pine Nuts and Garlic 65

Recipe 24: Air-Fried Jumbo Shrimp with Lime and Garlic 67

Recipe 25: Stuffed Chicken 69

Recipe 26: Beef Liver Skillet with Green Pepper . 71

Recipe 27: Beef and Sweet Potato Skillet 73

Recipe 28: Stuffed Pork 75

Recipe 29: Baked Talipa with Lemon and Mushrooms 78

Recipe 30: Salmon with Orange Sauce 80

CHAPTER 9: KETOGENIC DIET SNACKS AND SIDES 82

Recipe 31: Beet Salad 82

Recipe 32: Sweet Potato Fritters 84

Recipe 33: Eggplant Fries 86

Recipe 34: Sweet Potato Mash 88

Recipe 35: Cauliflower Sticks 90

Recipe 36: Southern-Style Salad 92

Recipe 37: Onion Fries 94

Recipe 38: Fried Spinach with Cashew Cream ... 96

Recipe 39: Stir-Fried Garlicky Mushrooms 98

Recipe 40: Gluten-Free Tortillas 100

CHAPTER 10: KETOGENIC DIET DINNER RECIPES 102

Recipe 41: Beef Picadillo 102

Recipe 42: Chicken Fajitas 105

Recipe 43: Teriyaki Burgers with Pineapple Salsa 107

Recipe 44: Spaghetti Squash 110

Recipe 45: Beef Roll 112

Recipe 46: Beef Meatballs with Sweet Potato Mash 114

Recipe 47: Glazed Meatloaf 117

Recipe 48: Bacon Stuffed Beef Mignon 119

Recipe 49: Tuna Salad 121

Recipe 50: Shrimp Salad 123

CHAPTER 11: KETOGENIC DIET DESSERT RECIPES 125

Recipe 51: Almond Cookies 125

Recipe 52: Caramel Flan 127

Recipe 53: Chocolate Chia Cookies 129

Recipe 54: Sesame Crackers 131

Recipe 55: Cocoa Truffles 133

Recipe 56: Gluten-Free Tiramisu 134

Recipe 57: Oven Baked Apples 136

Recipe 58: Avocado and Chocolate Mousse 138

Recipe 59: Chocolate Brownies 139

Recipe 60: Zucchini, Chocolate Bread 141

CHAPTER 12: CONCLUSION 143

INTRODUCTION

If you have been on a restless quest of losing weight and get your body into shape, then you have taken the same long path as me. I am not exaggerating when I say I tried all sorts of healthy diets that I have heard of so far; I kept taking all types of pills in order to lose weight, but everything failed and I woke up as early as birds to walk, exercise to lose weight.

I would spend long hours exercising; and I was over the moon when I discovered that I lost several pounds. And guess what? I didn't lose any pound and surprisingly enough, I figured out that I gained more weight instead. It was then when I found out that it was the right time for a life change. Hence, I made my decision and adopted the Ketogenic diet. And on this framework, I offer you this cookbook entitled: *"The Complete Ketogenic Diet Cookbook. Your Essential Keto Guide With Easy and Budget-Friendly Recipes For Weight Loss and Body Health."*

If you want to know more about the Ketogenic diet, then let me tell you that the Ketogenic Diet is said to be the diet of the century and it has been inspiring scientists to develop a more sophisticated and organized lifestyle that high promises in preventing certain serious diseases like cancer. Yet, the Ketogenic diet is not a magic spell; but it can be extremely effective in helping you step towards the process of losing weight without exhausting your body.

What is special about the Ketogenic diet is that it is known for its ability to get your body in the process of metabolism early and it will pretty much give you the health advantages you are seeking if you want to lose weight. And this diet has proven its ability to strengthen your heart and boosts your energy level to be able to work and cope with your everyday challenges and activities.

So if you are experiencing any sort of health issues and you have been feeling bad and unhealthy recently; this cookbook is for you! If you have also lost control over your weight and you have lost your hope, don't panic and don't worry about your health anymore because this Ketogenic cookbook will be your best guide from now on. If you are wondering what you are going to learn in this book, then here is a quick preview:

- The Ketogenic diet etymology
- The history of the Ketogenic diet
- The benefits of adopting the Ketogenic diet
- A large array of Ketogenic recipes

I hope that what you are going to learn about the Ketogenic diet from this cookbook, will help you enjoy its healthy benefits. Consequently, you will get used to a new, but balanced diet that will change your entire life forever with the versatility of its recipes and the easy-to follow recipes and directions.

Buckle up because your Ketogenic journey is about to start!

CHAPTER 2: KETOGENIC DIET, ETYMOLOGY

When scientists talk about diets, we tend to believe that the main objective of any diet aims at losing weight; however, it is not always the case. Indeed, the use of a diet can be an effective prescription to deal with a specific health conditions like arthritis and other diseases.

One of the most well – known dietary programs is the Ketogenic diet. The history of the Ketogenic diet dates back to the therapy of epilepsy of the nineteen twenties and the thirties. It was also used in order to be an alternative substitute for what was called the non – mainstream fasting.

And studies have demonstrated that Ketogenic diets worked very well as an epileptic therapy. Nevertheless, the Ketogenic diet was completely abandoned after creating many anticonvulsant therapies. Yet, despite the newly-introduced, developed therapies, scientists revealed in many studies that even developed medications failed to control epilepsy in more than 30% of the epileptic conditions and most of them were in children. Ketogenic diets were the only effective programs that proved its unrivalled success in controlling epilepsy. But what is epilepsy?

Epilepsy can be defined as a neurological disorder that may affect people in different stages of their lives. It also means a frequent number of seizure problems that are most of the times unpredictable. The severity of the seizure varies from a person to the other and trying any wrong method to control it may result in worsening the patient's condition and causing unpredicted neurological problems.

It is a condition that affects people's safety as well as their daily habits and even social relations and the only successful medium to control it is 100% dietary. In, fact the role of eating habits interfered with the treatment of epilepsy with the introduction of the fasting concept into mankind thousands of years ago. So what does the word "Ketogenic" mean?

The word Ketogenic is derived from ketosis. Ketosis is a pathological condition and a metabolic status during which the human body produces ketones in order to be used as fuel by specific organs that need glycogen to function. This exact condition happens, especially, during starvations and fasting.
A good Ketogenic diet is generally made up of the elements below:

- A high presence of healthy fats
- A balanced level of protein within the human body.
- A low level of carbohydrates

What happens exactly in a Ketogenic diet is that it causes the body to produce ketones. Indeed, during a Ketogenic diet, the primal source of the provided energy is fat and when it is combined with reduced consumption of carbohydrates, the body produces ketones.

When we follow a regular Ketogenic diet, the food we eat is transformed into glucose; then is transported around our bodies to be used as a source of energy, mainly by the brain. Our brain relies on the use of glucose as its source of energy; yet when the quantity of carbohydrates is very low, the liver starts processing fats in order to provide the brain with the energy it needs and these fats are called fatty acids and ketone elements.

If the level of ketone elements increases, it leads to ketosis. Many studies have shown that following a Ketogenic diet reduces the seizures especially in children. What characterizes the classic Ketogenic diet is that the ratio of fats to proteins and carbohydrates make together 4:1. We can mention many examples of fatty foods like cream, butter, olive oil, lard, duck fat. There are also a variety of foods high in carbohydrates we should avoid like pasta, sugar, grains; starchy fruits and so on.

CHAPTER 3: BACKGROUND AND HISTORY OF THE KETOGENIC DIET

The concept of Ketogenic diet originates from fasting; indeed, it was a dietary regime developed by physicians in order to mimic it. It all started in 1921when the Mayo Clinic was passing through a critical point as physicians tried to come up with new dietary solutions that can be as successful as fasting in treating epilepsy.

Many breakthroughs and discussions were witnessed when a doctor suggested applying The Ketogenic diet as an alternative to capture the same effects of fasting. And if we look back at history, we will find that the human kind had always suffered from epilepsy since the primitive stages of life on earth. However, due to illiteracy and due to the ignorance of humans at all the levels, people used to believe that epilepsy was rather due to the presence of supernatural effects of evil spirits.

The legend of epilepsy as an evil attack was only changed with Hippocrates, the Greek Physician. Hippocrates was the first to declare that Epilepsy was a biological rather than an evil spiritual illness and Hippocrates was the first to discover that fasting was the only means to control that illness. Hippocrates wasn't the only physician mentioned in history; many other physicians were also unfolded after him. And thanks to the hard work and

14

continuous experiments as well as research, Ketogenic diet found its way to the daily dietary habits of people around the globe. The breakthrough of the Ketogenic diet might have taken place exactly at the beginning of the twentieth century, when Marie and Guelpa, two French doctors helped around twenty people in minimizing the effects of their own epileptic conditions and recorded their healing process in a detailed report. And after a short time, similar experiences and conclusions were found and revealed in the United States when a number of doctors experimented fasting in order to improve the health conditions of their patients.

And to better understand the gradual transition from the fasting method to the dieting method, it is crucial to find out the connecting thread between them. The scientist William Lennox, who belonged to Harvard's Medical school, dedicated his life to studying the relationship between dieting and fasting. William Lenox found out that seizures started subsiding after around three days. He deduced that after following a specific Ketogenic diet, the human body started fuelling itself on its fat. And it was in the year 1921 that Dr. Rollin Woodyatt, an endocrinologist, found out that the beta-hydroxybutyric and acetone were two elements that were found in patients who followed a specific diet high in fats and low in carbohydrates. And beta- hydroxybutyric and acetone are known for belonging to the Ketogenic family. And later Dr. Wilder suggested that the human body can produce similar ketone elements within our blood similar to the elements produced in fasting. And with this discovery, Wilder gave the new diet a name and called it the Ketogenic diet.

As the Ketogenic diet positively impacted the human body, it soon became an unquestionable weapon in the medical fight against Epilepsy. The efficacy of the Ketogenic diet was proved on the practical level within the industry of pharmacology starting from 1938 when the first antiepileptic drugs were finally released to the market. And over the following thirty years, Ketogenic diet started to spread out to allow epileptic patients to live their lives without the need to adhere to a severe and a very strict dietary regime.

Later, in 1971, and oil diet was developed. Scientists tried to discover more properties of the Ketogenic diet so that it wouldn't be consecrated to epileptic patients. And it took a few years to develop the Ketogenic diet and to prove that it is not only a medicinal dieting method, but rather an entire style of life.

CHAPTER 4: BENEFITS OF ADOPTING A KETOGENIC DIET

The Ketogenic diet has numerous benefits that can be noticed since the first month of following it. Here are some of the benefits of a Ketogenic diet:

1. Weight loss

The most immediate benefit of the Ketogenic diet is the rapid weight loss that is primary achieves in obese diabetics. This is because reducing obesity can bring down a variety of other health problems that have been caused by it. One of the biggest benefits of this diet is that it can suppress appetite and long-term hunger. This can be helpful in case people are obese because of food addiction and will also prevent weight gain in the future.

2. Increase in healthy cholesterol

Indeed, the Ketogenic diet reduces the consumption of carbohydrates, but stimulates the consumption of saturated fats; the levels of good cholesterol will go higher. A healthier heart can be induced by these levels of healthy cholesterols.

3. Reduction of triglycerides and sugar levels

Triglyceride levels and carbohydrate consumption have a direct relationship; when one falls, the other does too. The risk of heart attack can be reduced in this way. The levels of sugar and insulin also fall. The blood sugar and insulin levels will no longer be increased because there will be less sugar.

4. Controls blood pressure
When the consumption of carbohydrates is reduced, the control of the blood pressure becomes easier. You can also stop taking blood pressure medications because it gradually reaches a normal level if the Ketogenic diet is strictly followed.

5. Reduces the levels of cholesterol
Excess glucose in the regular diet leads to the production of cholesterol in the body. When the number of sugar-creating foods is reduced, your arterial system is not damaged and the inflammation decreases. As the level of glucose in the blood decreases, the cholesterol level also decreases.

6. Pain Reliever

The reduction of joint pain and stiffness is certainly another benefit of this diet. A Ketogenic diet is the reason why cereal-based foods are removed from your daily diet. These foods are the main cause of pain and chronic disease and these problems will automatically disappear.

7. Improves the quality of sleep
Improving sleep habits is another benefit of the Ketogenic diet. Sleep apnoea and other sleep disorders are caused by grain consumption and their elimination can lead to better sleep habits. You have to give up on having your favourite snacks for a while.

8. Improves digestion

Food will be digested very quickly, resulting in decreased gas, bloating and stomach pain. The consumption of cereals and sugar is the cause of these problems, and their elimination will be healthy. Again, sugar and grains can cause heartburn problems that will eventually disappear once these foods are removed from the diet.

9. Boosts energy

Chronic fatigue symptoms disappear automatically when a Ketogenic diet is adopted. Experience better energy levels with higher levels of energy due to changing foods.

CHAPTER 5: WHAT TO EAT AND WHAT NOT TO EAT ON A KETOGENIC DIET

If you have recently adopted the Ketogenic diet, you should first learn the main basics of this diet, and you have to know what to eat and what not to eat on this diet. And on that note, here is a list of what you can eat and what you should avoid on a Ketogenic diet.

What you can eat on a Ketogenic diet

- Almond butter and coconut cream: Make sure to look for grass-fed natural products wherever is possible

- The consumption of cheeses should be moderate: Like Cheddar cheese, Blue cheese, feta cheese, whole white cheese, mozzarella, whole milk ricotta cheese and Gruyere cheese, but goat cheese is always the best choice for the Ketogenic diet.

- Eggs: if possible use raised outdoors eggs because they contain more omega-3

- Other ingredients like dark chocolate and cocoa powder, coffee, and unsweetened tea.

- Nuts and seeds in moderation: Walnuts, almonds, pumpkin seeds, flax seeds, and Chia seeds.

- Vegetable oils in moderation: Basically, extra virgin olive oil, coconut oil, linseed oil, fish oil.

- Tomatoes, onions and peppers

- Low sugar fruits: blueberries, lemon, raspberries, strawberries.

- The Ketogenic diet allows the use of salt, pepper and other spices and herbs
- Meat: Ham, red meat, bacon, sausages, turkey and chicken.
- Greasy fish: Like salmon, trout, seafood, mackerel, and tuna.
- Almond flour
- Coconut flour
- Gluten ingredients
- Sugar
- Soy
- All types of packaged snacks
- White breads
- Amaranth
- Pasta

What not to eat on Foods to avoid

Stay away from Sweet foods: Like soda, cream, cakes, sweets smoothies, fruit juice, and ice-cream.

- Legumes like beans, peas, lentils and chickpeas.
- Starches or cereals and all other flour-based products like wheat
- Root like potatoes, carrots and parsnips.

- Avoid all types of Alcohol because of its high carbohydrate content and numerous alcoholic drinks can prevent you from reaching the state of ketosis.
- Stay away from bananas and high-carbohydrate ingredients.

Note

Always make sure to check the food labels because that is important to know the count of calories and carbohydrates you are using.

Useful Abbreviations of Units Used In the Recipes

- 1 lb ....1 pound
- 1 Oz ....1 ounce
- 1Tbsp 1tablespoon
- 1 Tsp 1teaspoon
- The list of Nutrient use these abbreviations:
- 1 g ....1 gram
- 1 mg ....1 milligram

CHAPTER 6: KETOGENIC DIET BREAKFAST RECIPES

Recipe 1: Chocolate Chia Pudding

(Prep time: 5 minutes\ Cook Time: 10 minutes\ Servings: 3)

INGREDIENTS

- 2 Tablespoons of chia seeds
- 450 ml Water
- 1 Cup of Whey chocolate protein
- 1 Greek, sugar-free Yogurt
- ½ Cup of Roasted linseeds
- 1 Tablespoon of unsweetened cocoa powder
- Stevia (optional)

Directions:

1. Mix the chia seeds with water and let stand for 20 minutes. Stir occasionally.
2. Once the chia seeds are well inflated, add all the other ingredients and mix again.
3. Put for about 30 minutes in the fridge before serving.

Nutrition facts
Amount per Serving
Calories- 188 g.
Fats- 12 g.
Fibre- 1.6g.
Carbohydrate- 3 g.
Protein- 15g.

The nutritional details are in general estimate and they should only be used like a guide with approximate use

Recipe 2: Sweet potato Muffins

(Prep time: 10 minutes\ Cook Time: 30 minutes\ Servings: 6-7)

INGREDIENTS:

- 1 ¼ cups sweet potato, finely chopped
- 3 TBSP white Onion, diced
- 1 tsp red onion, finely chopped
- 3 1/3 heap cups spinach, finely chopped
- 5 Large eggs, pasteurized
- 5 Large egg whites
- ¼ Cup coconut milk
- 2 tsp fresh chives, finely chopped
- ½ tsp, extra virgin olive oil
- ¾ clove garlic, finely minced
- 1 Pinch nutmeg
- 1 Pinch salt
- 1 Pinch pepper

Directions:

1. Start by preheating your oven to about 400 degrees Fahrenheit.
2. Lightly spray a standard muffin tin with cooking spray
3. In a large bowl; whisk all together the egg whites, coconut milk, and chives; then whisk the mixture and season with 1 pinch of salt and 1 pinch of pepper

4. Heat the oil in a large pan and over medium high heat; then add in the sweet potatoes and the chopped onion
5. Cook the mixture for about 7 to 8 minutes; then add the spinach, nutmeg and garlic and cook for 2 additional minutes
6. Once the spinach becomes wilted, remove the pan from the heat and set it aside to cool for about 2 minutes; then crack the pasteurized eggs into a small bowl and add it to the mixture
7. Combine your mixture very well; then pour the obtained batter into the muffin tin and make sure that to pour an even mixture into each of the muffin cups
8. Bake the muffins for about 18 to 20 minutes
9. Serve and enjoy your breakfast muffins immediately!

Nutrition facts
Amount per Serving
Calories- 132 g.
Fats- 6.3 g.
Fibre- 1.6g.
Carbohydrate- 8.5g.
Protein- 12g.

The nutritional details are in general estimate and they should only be used like a guide with approximate use

Recipe 3: Granola Bars

(Prep time: 10 minutes\ Cook Time: 25 minutes\ Servings: 6)

INGREDIENTS

- 2 cups of flaxseed oatmeal
- 1/2 cup of organic coconut oil
- 1/2 cup of organic agave syrup
- 1/2 cup grated coconut
- 1/4 cup of cocoa
- Crumbled hazelnuts

Directions:

1. Preheat your oven to 150 degrees
2. Mix all ingredients in a large container
3. Spread out your mixture in a compact way on a baking sheet.
4. Cook for 25 minutes at 150 degrees. To form large nuggets, flip after the first 10 minutes
5. Serve and enjoy your breakfast!

Nutrition facts
Amount per Serving
Calories- 132 g.
Fats- 6.3 g.
Fibre- 1.6g.
Carbohydrate- 8.5g.
Protein- 12g.

The nutritional details are in general estimate and they should only be used like a guide with approximate use

Recipe 4: Mushroom Quiche

(Prep time: 9 minutes\ Cook Time: 30 minutes\ Servings: 5)

INGREDIENTS:

- 1 lb breakfast grass-fed turkey sausage
- 1 Small onion, finely chopped
- 5 Cups spinach, roughly chopped
- 2 Cups mushrooms, thinly sliced
- 2 Thinly sliced tomatoes
- ½ Cup coconut milk, full fat
- 11 to12 pasteurized large eggs
- 1 Pinch salt
- 1 Pinch black pepper, freshly ground
- ¼ tsp garlic powder

Directions:

1. Preheat the oven to about 400° Fahrenheit.
2. Finely slice the mushrooms, then chop the onion
3. Heat a large pan over medium heat or you can just use an iron skillet
4. Add in the onion and the sausage and stir from time to time for about 7 minutes
5. Add in the sliced mushrooms and cook for a couple of minutes; then remove the skillet or pan from the heat
6. Finely chop the spinach and crack the eggs into a bowl, one by one; then add in the coconut milk

7. Whisk the ingredients all together very well; then add in the spinach, the garlic powder, salt and pepper
8. Whisk again until you get a light mixture; then add the sausage to your mixture with the remaining ingredients and mix
9. Spray a 9x9 oven safe square dish with cooking spray
10. Pour the mixture into the pan and top with the sliced tomatoes
11. Bake in the preheated oven for about 30 minutes or until the top gets a brown color and crispy texture
12. Once perfectly baked, remove the pan from the oven and set it aside for about 5 minutes to cool down
13. Slice the quiche into even pieces; then serve and enjoy your delicious breakfast!

Nutrition facts
Amount per Serving
Calories- 281 g.
Fats- 20 g.
Fibre- 1.2g.
Carbohydrate- 2.4g.
Protein- 18g.
The nutritional details are in general estimate and they should only be used like a guide with approximate use

Recipe 5: Almond Flour Pancakes

(Prep time: 10 minutes\ Cook Time: 15 minutes\ Servings: 4)

INGREDIENTS:

- 1 1/4 cups Coconut Milk, full fat
- 1/3 Cup Tapioca Flour
- 1/3 Cup Almond Flour
- 1 tsp sea salt
- ½ tsp turmeric powder
- 1 tsp Chilli Powder
- ½ Small red onion, finely diced
- ¼ tsp black pepper, freshly ground
- A few cilantro leaves, roughly chopped
- 1 Medium Serrano pepper, finely minced
- ¼Inch ginger, finely grated
- 2 TBSP Extra virgin olive oil or coconut oil, melted

Directions:

1. Start by making the batter and to do that, take a large bowl
2. Add the tapioca flour, almond flour and the spices to the bowl and give the mixture a good stir
3. Add in the cilantro, Serrano pepper, ginger and onion

4. Make sure your batter is smooth and everything perfectly combined
5. Heat a medium sauté pan on medium-low heat; then in the 2 tablespoons of oil
6. Pour about ¼ cup of the batter into the pan and gently spread it into the pan
7. Fry for about 3 minutes per side; and if you notice the sides are getting brown quickly, drizzle a little quantity of oil before you flip the pancake
8. Remove the pancake to a serving plate and repeat the same process with the remaining batter
9. Serve and enjoy your succulent pancakes!

Nutrition facts

Amount per Serving

Calories- 192 g.

Fats- 10.5 g.

Fibre- 1.3g.

Carbohydrate- 8.3g.

Protein- 5.7g.

The nutritional details are in general estimate and they should only be used like a guide with approximate use

Recipe 6: Cashew Pudding

(Prep time: 3 minutes\ Cook Time: 5 minutes\ Servings: 3)

INGREDIENTS:

- 2 Cups cashews
- 2 Small dates
- 5 TBSP Chia seeds
- 2 ½ Cups cold water
- 3 ½ Hemp seeds
- ¼ tsp cinnamon
- 1 pinch sea salt

For the toppings:

- Chopped dried or fresh fruits
- Chopped pecans or walnuts
- 2 TBSP sunflower seeds

Directions:

1. Place the cashews, dates and hemp seeds in a blender; then pour the water over the nuts and blend on high speed for about 1 minute
2. Pour in 2 additional cups of water; then add the cinnamon, salt and Chia seeds and pulse until your mixture is combined; if the pudding is too thick, you can add the remaining ½ cup of water
3. Refrigerate the pudding for about 1 hour

4. Top with the nuts and fresh fruits
5. Serve and enjoy your delicious pudding!

Nutrition facts

Amount per Serving

Calories- 153 g.

Fats- 8.95 g.

Fibre- 3.1 g.

Carbohydrate- 12.3 g.

Protein- 6 g.

The nutritional details are in general estimate and they should only be used like a guide with approximate use

Recipe 7: Breakfast Omelette

(Prep time: 3 minutes\ Cook Time: 6 minutes\ Servings: 2)

INGREDIENTS

- 2 eggs
- 1 tbsp coconut oil
- 1 Cup of Tomatoes
- 2 Tablespoons of goat cheese
- 1 Cup of coconut milk
- Season according to your taste

Directions

1. Heat the pan and add a little coconut oil.
2. Beat the eggs with 1 tablespoon milk, salt, pepper and the remaining spices.
3. Pour the mixture into the pan.
4. Slice the tomatoes and feta into cubes and place on the omelette in the pan.
5. Reduce to medium heat and watch the omelette cooking for about 6 minutes.
6. The omelet is ready when the bottom begins to turn into brown and the feta is melted.

Nutrition facts
Amount per Serving
Calories- 340 g.
Fats- 27 g.
Fibre- 1.9 g.
Carbohydrate- 1.7 g.
Protein- 21 g.

The nutritional details are in general estimate and they should only be used like a guide with approximate use

Recipe 8: Gluten Free Bread

(Prep time: 15 minutes\ Cook Time: 60 minutes\ Servings: 4)

INGREDIENTS:

- 2 Large eggs, beaten
- ¼ Cup coconut oil, melted
- ¼ Cup apple butter, unsweetened
- 2 Cups sifted almond flour
- 2 Cups assorted hazelnuts, almonds and cashews
- 2 Cups chopped dried fruits
- 1 tsp baking powder
- 1 Pinch salt

Directions:

1. Set the oven to about 350°F temperature
2. Spray a standard medium, 9" x 5" loaf pan with cooking spray
3. Line the loaf pan with a parchment paper and set it aside
4. Crack the eggs in a large mixing bowl and add the coconut oil and the apple butter; then combine very well
5. Add the salt and the baking powder and mix again
6. Add in the nuts and the fruits and whisk with a spatula

7. Pour the batter into the loaf pan and make sure it is smooth on top
8. Lay a little piece of aluminium foil over the loaf pan to prevent from browning
9. Place the loaf pan in the oven and bake for about 60 minutes; remove the foil during the last 9 minutes
10. Once baked, remove the loaf pan from the oven and lift the gluten-free bread and place it over a rack to cool for 4 minutes
11. Slice your gluten-free bread with a sharp knife; then serve and enjoy!

Nutrition facts

Amount per Serving

Calories- 323 g.

Fats- 24 g.

Fibre- 2.02 g.

Carbohydrate- 12 g.

Protein- 9.8 g.

The nutritional details are in general estimate and they should only be used like a guide with approximate use

Recipe 9: Egg Roll

(Prep time: 10 minutes\ Cook Time: 20 minutes\ Servings: 3)

INGREDIENTS:

- 2 TBSP ghee
- 1 Medium carrot, peeled and grated
- 1 Pinch sea salt
- 2 Cloves garlic, finely minced
- 5 Large pasteurized eggs
- 1 Medium red onion, thinly sliced
- 1 Small white onion, thinly sliced
- 1 Pinch black pepper, freshly ground
- 1 TBSP Coconut oil
- 1 TBSP mayonnaise
- 2 Slices free range ham

Directions:

1. Preheat the oven to a temperature of about 350 °F.
2. Heat the ghee in a medium heavy skillet; then add in the onion and sauté for about 4 minutes
3. Add in the grated carrot; then sprinkle with 1 pinch of salt and cook for about 5 minutes; make sure to stir from time to time to prevent burning and cook for 4 additional minutes

4. Add in the garlic with 1 pinch of salt and 1 pinch of pepper right by the end
5. Crack the eggs with 1 pinch salt in a bowl and whisk very well
6. Put a large parchment paper in an 8-9 by 14-15 oven tray and lightly spray with melted coconut oil or ghee
7. Pour in the egg batter and quickly tuck away the baking paper into its corners to make sure the batter won't escape from the corners
8. Pour the mixture of onion and carrots on top and spread it very well
9. Place the baking pan in the oven and bake for about 16 to 17 minutes
10. Remove the baking tray from the oven and carefully lift the baking paper
11. Place the over a cutting board and spread a little bit of mayonnaise and scattered ham
12. Without removing the baking paper, start rolling from the base and fold inwards the egg roll until you finish
13. Remove the paper off and slice the rolled egg; then serve and enjoy your delicious breakfast!

Nutrition facts
Amount per Serving
Calories- 150 g.
Fats- 10 g.
Fibre- 2.7 g.
Carbohydrate- 10.1 g.
Protein- 8 g.

The nutritional details are in general estimate and they should only be used like a guide with approximate use

Recipe 10: Sweet Potato Waffles

(Prep time: 15 minutes\ Cook Time: 20 minutes\ Servings: 5)

INGREDIENTS:

- 2 Medium sweet potatoes, peeled and grated
- 3 Medium eggs, beaten large
- 1 tsp cinnamon
- 1 Pinch salt
- 1 Pinch black pepper
- 1 tsp red pepper flakes
- 1 tsp garlic powder
- 1 TBSP Coconut oil, for greasing the waffle iron with

Directions:

1. Preheat a waffle iron on medium high heat
2. Combine the sweet potatoes with the cinnamon, eggs, sea salt, red pepper flakes, garlic powder and black pepper in a large bowl and mix until all the ingredients are very well combined
3. The waffle iron should be already hot by now, so lightly grease both the bottom and top of its inside
4. Ladle about 1/3rd of the egg and sweet potato mixture into your waffle iron

5. Push the mixture into a circular shape all the way to the waffle edge and cook for about 16 to 18 minutes

6. Wait for about 2 minutes; then gently turn off the waffle iron

7. Serve and enjoy your sweet potato waffles

Nutrition facts
Amount per Serving
Calories- 119 g.
Fats- 2.1 g.
Fibre- 1.9 g.
Carbohydrate- 11 g.
Protein- 5.3 g.

The nutritional details are in general estimate and they should only be used like a guide with approximate use

CHAPTER 7: KETOGENIC DIET APPETIZERS

Recipe 11: Cauliflower Muffins

(Prep time: 5 minutes\ Cook Time: 20 minutes\ Servings: 6)

INGREDIENTS:

- Half a head of cauliflower
- 2 Cups of mushrooms
- 6 Organic eggs
- 2 Tablespoons of fresh coconut milk
- 1 Minced garlic clove
- 2 teaspoons of chopped chives
- 2 tablespoons of coconut oil, melted
- 1 Cup of grated goat cheese
- Salt and pepper

Directions:

1. Steam cauliflower, cool and crush with a fork.
2. Fry the minced mushrooms in the butter. Mix with the rest of the ingredients and put in muffin pans.

3. Bake for 20 minutes in the oven at 180 °C/360° F. The muffins should be golden brown.

4. Serve and enjoy your muffins

Nutrition facts

Amount per Serving

Calories- 288 g.

Fats- 17.8 g.

Fibre- 0.9 g.

Carbohydrate- 6 g.

Protein- 18 g.

The nutritional details are in general estimate and they should only be used like a guide with approximate use

Recipe 12: Stuffed Sardines

(Prep time: 15 minutes\ Cook Time: 30 minutes\ Servings: 7)

INGREDIENTS:

- 1 lb sardines, raw and fresh
- 2 TBSP yellow raisins, soaked in water
- 2 TBSP pine nuts, chopped
- 2 Anchovies, finely minced
- 1 TBSP almond flour
- ½ TBSP flat leaf parsley, minced
- ½ orange, juiced
- 1 Medium lemon, sliced
- 1 Pinch salt
- 1 Pinch black pepper, freshly ground
- 2 TBSP coconut oil
- ½ Cup black olives, hulled and chopped
- 2 Bay leaves

Directions:

1. Clean the sardines and rinse very well; then carefully remove the spines with a sharp knife or with your hands
2. Set the sardines aside
3. Melt the 2 tablespoons of coconut oil in a large and heavy non-stick frying pan

4. Add the anchovies and the almond milk and sauté over medium high heat for about 3 minutes; then set aside to cool
5. Mix the toasted almond and anchovies with the pine nuts, black olive, salt, raisins and pepper; then stir
6. Preheat the oven to about 390° F
7. Grease a baking tray with cooking spray and arrange the sardines with the side up in the tray and place about 1 teaspoon of the filling in each of the sardines
8. Cover each sardine with another sardine with the spine removed
9. Drizzle with the lemon juice and bake for about 20 minutes
10. Remove the tray from the oven when the time is up and set aside to cool for 3 minutes
11. Serve and enjoy your dish with lemon sliced and top with chopped parsley!

Nutrition facts
Amount per Serving
Calories- 342 g.
Fats- 13.7 g.
Fibre- 2.1 g.
Carbohydrate- 11 g.
Protein- 14.5 g.

The nutritional details are in general estimate and they should only be used like a guide with approximate use

Recipe 13: Spring Roll Bowl

(Prep time: 5 minutes\ Cook Time: 25 minutes\ Servings: 4)

INGREDIENTS:

- 3 TBSP coconut oil, divided
- 1 Medium onion, diced
- 1 lb chicken, ground
- 3 Cloves garlic, finely minced
- 2 tsp chilli powder
- 1 tsp salt
- ½ tsp black pepper, ground
- 1 Medium bell pepper, diced
- ½ tsp cayenne
- ½ lb Brussels sprouts, finely shredded

Directions:

1. Melt about 2 tablespoons of coconut oil into a large non-stick, over medium high heat
2. Add in the onion and sauté for about 5 minutes
3. Add in the ground turkey, spices and garlic; then cook for about 15 minutes
4. Set a quantity of ground chicken meat aside in a dish, to create a space for the Brussels sprouts

5. Add the remaining tablespoon of coconut oil; then add in the Brussels sprouts and the bell pepper and sauté for about 4 minutes
6. Add in the meat that you have set aside and mix very well
7. Transfer the cooked mixture to a serving platter
8. Serve and enjoy your snack!

Nutrition facts

Amount per Serving

Calories- 320 g.

Fats- 19.3 g.

Fibre- 3.1 g.

Carbohydrate- 13 g.

Protein- 25 g.

The nutritional details are in general estimate and they should only be used like a guide with approximate use

Recipe 14: Stuffed Mushrooms

(Prep time: 10 minutes \ Cook Time: 30 minutes \ Servings: 7)

INGREDIENTS:

- 1 ½ lbs Baby Bella mushrooms, stems removed
- 1 lb Blue Crab Meat, finely shredded
- ¼ Cup Mayonnaise
- 3 ½ TBSP Chives, finely chopped
- ½ tsp Paprika
- ½ tsp oregano, dried

Directions:

1. Combine the shredded crab with the mayonnaise, the chives and the spices in a large bowl
2. Set the mixture aside for about 15 minutes; then preheat the oven to about 350° F
3. Clean the Bella mushrooms and make sure to remove the stems; then pat it dry with clean paper towels
4. Stuff the mushroom caps with the shredded crab mixture; then place it over a baking sheet lined with a large parchment paper
5. Bake the stuffed mushrooms for about 18 minutes
6. Remove the stuffed mushrooms from the oven and let rest for 2 minutes

7. Serve and enjoy your stuffed mushrooms!

Nutrition facts

Amount per Serving

Calories- 103.2 g.

Fats- 7.6 g.

Fibre- 0.6 g.

Carbohydrate- 2.6 g.

Protein- 6.4 g.

*The nutritional details are in general estimate and they
should only be used like a guide with approximate use*

Recipe 15: Roasted Cauliflower

(Prep time: 6 minutes\ Cook Time: 27 minutes\ Servings: 5)

INGREDIENTS:

- 2 Small heads broccoli
- 1 TBSP olive oil
- 1 Pinch salt
- 1 tsp coconut oil, melted
- 3 TBSP pine nuts
- 1 Pinch Chile flakes

Directions:

1. Preheat the oven to about 425° F and line a baking sheet with a parchment paper
2. Cut each of the broccoli heads into halves; then carefully cut each of the halves again
3. Put the broccoli over a baking sheet with the side down and season with the salt and drizzle with the olive oil
4. Sprinkle a little bit of salt on top again and bake in the oven for about 20 minutes
5. Remove the broccoli from the oven and flip; then bake for about 5 additional minutes
6. In the meantime, melt the coconut in a frying pan over medium high heat; then add the pine nuts and sauté for about 2 minutes and shake from time to time

7. Remove the broccoli from the oven and transfer it to a serving platter
8. Sprinkle the pine nuts on top and garnish with the chilli flakes
9. Serve and enjoy!

Nutrition facts

Amount per Serving

Calories- 126 g.

Fats- 9.9 g.

Fibre- 2.2 g.

Carbohydrate- 8 g.

Protein- 5.8 g.

The nutritional details are in general estimate and they should only be used like a guide with approximate use

Recipe 16: Stuffed Peppers

(Prep time: 8 minutes\ Cook Time: 10 minutes\ Servings: 7)

INGREDIENTS:

- 7 Large bell peppers, green or red
- 1 lb ground beef
- 1 tsp garlic salt
- 1 tsp basil, finely chopped
- ¼ tsp black pepper
- 1 Large egg, lightly beaten
- ¼ Cup coconut flour
- 2 ½ TBSP olive oil

Directions:

1. Start by cutting the tops off the bell peppers and remove the seeds; then set the peppers aside
2. In a large mixing bowl, combine the ground beef with the garlic salt, the egg, the coconut flour, the Italian seasoning, the basil and the pepper
3. Stuffed the peppers with the mixture; then heat a large skillet over medium high heat and spray it with olive oil
4. When the oil heats up, arrange the peppers and cook for about 4 minutes; then flip the

pepper and cook it for about 3 additional minutes on the other side
5. Remove the stuffed peppers from the skillet and transfer it to a serving platter
6. Serve and enjoy your stuffed peppers!

Nutrition facts

Amount per Serving

Calories- 175 g.

Fats- 6 g.

Fibre- 1.3 g.

Carbohydrate- 10.7 g.

Protein- 5.8 g.

The nutritional details are in general estimate and they should only be used like a guide with approximate use

Recipe 17: Roasted Squash

(Prep time: 3 minutes\ Cook Time: 5 minutes\ Servings: 3)

INGREDIENTS:

- 1 Medium butternut squash, seeded, peeled and diced into cubes
- 3 TBSP extra-virgin olive oil
- 3 cloves garlic, finely minced
- 1/3 Cup, parsley, finely chopped
- 1 TBSP rosemary, chopped
- ¾ tsp salt
- ½ tsp black pepper, ground

Directions:

1. Bring a saucepan equipped with a steamer basket and filled with water to a boil
2. Add the squash to the steamer basket, then cover and steam both for about 13 minutes
3. Heat the oil in a small frying pan over medium high heat; then add the garlic and cook for about 3 minutes
4. Place the oil and garlic in a large bowl; then add the herbs and mix
5. Add the squash to the herb and garlic mixture; then season with the salt and salt and give a stir
6. Serve and enjoy your dish!

Nutrition facts

Amount per Serving

Calories- 99 g.

Fats- 5.7 g.

Fibre- 2.5 g.

Carbohydrate- 11 g.

Protein- 4 g.

The nutritional details are in general estimate and they should only be used like a guide with approximate use

Recipe 18: Chicken Fingers

(Prep time: 5 minutes\ Cook Time: 10 minutes\ Servings: 4)

INGREDIENTS:

- 1 lb chicken breast, chopped into chunks
- 3 TBSP arrowroot flour
- 2 tsp paprika
- ¾ tsp sea salt, unrefined
- ½ tsp onion powder
- ½ Cup Coconut oil

Directions:

1. Combine the paprika with the arrowroot flour, onion powder and salt in a small bowl
2. Toss each chicken piece into the flour mixture until it is very-well coated
3. Pour the coconut oil in a large frying pan over medium high heat and let it melt
4. When the coconut oil melts, add in the chicken
5. Fry the chicken pieces for about 3 minutes; then flip and fry for about 2 minutes
6. Remove the chicken nuggets from the skillet
7. Serve and enjoy your chicken nuggets!

Nutrition facts
Amount per Serving
Calories- 148 g.

Fats- 7 g.
Fibre- 0.1 g.
Carbohydrate- 11.2 g.
Protein- 15 g.

The nutritional details are in general estimate and they should only be used like a guide with approximate use

Recipe 19: Zucchini Fritters

(Prep time: 6 minutes\ Cook Time: 10 minutes\ Servings: 5-6)

INGREDIENTS:

- 2 Medium carrots, peeled and thinly diced
- 2 Medium zucchinis, shredded
- 1 Cup coconut flour
- 1 Large egg, beaten
- 1 Small white onion, finely chopped
- 1 Cup parsley, finely chopped
- ¾ Cups apples, finely chopped
- 3 TBS olive oil
- 1 Pinch sea salt
- 1 Pinch black pepper

Directions:

1. Shred the zucchini, the apples, the onions and the carrot with a veggie chopper
2. Wash the veggie in a colander and set it aside for about 5 minutes
3. Pat the veggies dry and squeeze to remove any remaining quantity of water
4. Put the veggies in a large bowl; then add in the egg, the flour and combine very well; then add the parsley and mix
5. Season with the salt and pepper

6. Warm the oil in a large pan over medium high heat
7. Form fritters of the mixture and when the oil is hot enough, drop the fritters into it and fry for about 2 minutes per side
8. Serve and enjoy your fritters

Nutrition facts

Amount per Serving

Calories- 144.6 g.

Fats- 6 g.

Fibre- 1 g.

Carbohydrate- 7.1 g.

Protein- 8.3 g.

The nutritional details are in general estimate and they should only be used like a guide with approximate use

Recipe 20: Cashew Hummus

(Prep time: 5 minutes\ Cook Time: 35 minutes\ Servings: 3)

INGREDIENTS:

- 2 Cups raw cashews, soaked for about 60 minutes
- 3 TBSP coconut oil
- 2 TBSP lime, juiced
- 1 TBSP water
- 1 TBSP parsley leaves, fresh and finely chopped
- 1 Medium head garlic, roasted

For the topping:

- 1 Cup sun dried tomatoes, finely chopped
- 1 TBSP flat parsley leaves, finely chopped
- 1 Pinch black pepper, freshly cracked
- 1 Pinch salt
- 1 Drizzle olive oil
- 2 TBSP raw cashews, chopped

Directions:

1. Begin by roasting the garlic head, after cutting it in half, drizzling it with olive, in a preheated oven on about 400° F for about 32 minutes

2. After the garlic is roasted, remove it from the oven and peel off the cloves
3. Combine the cashews with the coconut oil, water, lime juice, and the chopped parsley in a food processor and pulse for about 1 to 2 minutes or until the mixture becomes smooth
4. Add the garlic and pulse again until the mixture gets tender and smooth
5. Adjust the seasoning with salt and pepper; then transfer the pulsed mixture to a serving plate and top with the dried tomatoes, fresh parsley, olive oil and cashews
6. Serve and enjoy!

Nutrition facts
Amount per Serving
Calories- 142 g.
Fats- 12 g.
Fibre- 1.2 g.
Carbohydrate- 6 g.
Protein- 4.5 g.

The nutritional details are in general estimate and they should only be used like a guide with approximate use

CHAPTER 8: KETOGENIC DIET LUNCH RECIPES

Recipe 21: Cauliflower Pizza

(Prep time: 12 minutes\ Cook Time: 30 minutes\ Servings: 5-6)

INGREDIENTS

- 1/2 head of cauliflower
- 80g of parmesan cheese
- 2 pasteurized eggs
- 2 tablespoons of organic hempseed oil
- 1 teaspoon balsamic vinegar
- 1 mozzarella cheese ball
- 1 handful of basil leaves

Directions:

1. Rinse the cauliflower, separate the heads and mix them. Mix and work until you get a consistency close to rice.
2. Boil some water in a saucepan and cook cauliflower for about 5 minutes. Drain and let cool.
3. Spin chilled cauliflower in a nearby dish towel to let out as much water and liquid as possible. The goal is to get some kind of flour.
4. Add eggs and Parmesan to this mixture and mix well.

5. Spread cauliflower pizza dough on baking paper. Spread well in a disk and cook for about 15 minutes at 200 ° C in a preheated oven.
6. Meanwhile, wash and cut the cherry tomatoes in half. Add hempseed oil and balsamic vinegar. Season with salt and pepper.
7. Unravel the mozzarella ball by hand into pieces.
8. Remove the pizza dough from the oven, add the tomatoes and mozzarella and re-enter for 15 minutes.
9. Garnish with fresh basil. Serve very hot.

Nutrition facts
Amount per Serving
Calories- 287 g.
Fats- 22 g.
Fibre- 1.4 g.
Carbohydrate- 2.9 g.
Protein- 26 g.

The nutritional details are in general estimate and they should only be used like a guide with approximate use

Recipe 22: Chicken Kabobs with Chimichurri Sauce

(Prep time: 7 minutes\ Cook Time: 10 minutes\ Servings: 4)

INGREDIENTS

- 1 and ¼ pounds of cubed chicken or beef meat
- 1 Pinch of fresh ground pepper
- 1 and ¼ tsp of sea salt
- 1 large; diced red onion
- 17 to 18 cherry tomatoes
- Soaked bamboo skewers
- Coils for fire

To make the Chimichurri sauce

- 2 tbsp of finely chopped parsley
- 2 tbsp of chopped cilantro
- 2 tbsp of finely chopped red onions
- 1 Minced garlic clove
- 2 tbsp of sesame olive oil
- 2 tbsp of apple cider vinegar
- 1 tbsp of water
- ¼ tsp of sea salt
- 1/8 tsp of fresh black pepper
- 1/8 tsp of crushed red pepper flakes

Directions

1. Season your chicken with 1 pinch of salt and 1 pinch of pepper
2. To make the chimichurri, combine the vinegar, the red onion, the salt and the sesame oil and set it aside for about 5 minutes
3. Place the onions, the beef and the tomatoes into the skewers.
4. Place the skewers on the coal fire
5. Cook the skewers for 10 minutes each side
6. Remove when cooked
7. Serve and enjoy your kabobs with the chimichurri sauce!

Nutrition facts

Amount per Serving

Calories- 265 g.

Fats- 9.3 g.

Fibre- 1.4 g.

Carbohydrate- 4.32 g.

Protein- 32 g.

The nutritional details are in general estimate and they should only be used like a guide with approximate use

Recipe 23: Chicken with Pine Nuts and Garlic

(Prep time: 5 minutes\ Cook Time: 10 minutes\ Servings: 3-4)

INGREDIENTS:

- 3 Chicken breasts, medium
- 1 TBSP salt
- 1 TBSP black pepper, freshly ground
- 3 TBSP pine nuts, lightly toasted
- 2 ¼ Batches, garlic pesto, roasted

For the pesto

- 1 Cup basil leaves, fresh and finely chopped
- 1 Bulb, Garlic
- ½ Cup Pine Nuts
- 1 Medium lemon, juiced
- ¼ Cup extra virgin olive oil
- 1 Pinch salt
- 1 Pinch black pepper, freshly ground

Directions:

ROAST THE GARLIC:

1. Preheat the oven to about 375° Fahrenheit.
2. Peel the garlic without breaking the bulb
3. Remove the top of the bulb by cutting it off with a knife
4. Wrap the garlic bulb in the aluminium foil and bake at a temperature of about 375° F for 40 minutes

5. In the meantime, toast the pine nuts in a medium pan over medium high heat and stir from time to time for about 5 minutes
6. Once the garlic is roasted, remove it from the oven
7. Add the chopped basil, the roasted garlic, half the a tablespoon of olive oil; then add the toasted pine nut to a blender or a food processor
8. Pulse your ingredients for 30 seconds; then season with 1 pinch salt, 1 pinch pepper and add the remaining quantity of oil and pulse until the mixture becomes smooth

FOR THE CHICKEN:

1. Preheat the oven to about 400° F.
2. Arrange the chicken breasts over a large baking sheet and sprinkle with the salt and pepper and bake for about 40 minutes
3. Set the chicken aside to cool down; then chop it into cubes about ½ inch each
4. Combine the chicken with the pesto in a large bowl
5. Sprinkle more pine nuts; then serve and enjoy in lettuce leaves!

Nutrition facts
Amount per Serving
Calories- 204 g.
Fats- 8.5 g.
Fibre- 0.4 g.
Carbohydrate- 2.6 g.
Protein- 29 g.
The nutritional details are in general estimate and they should only be used like a guide with approximate use

Recipe 24: Air-Fried Jumbo Shrimp with Lime and Garlic

(Prep time: 7 minutes\ Cook Time: 15 minutes\ Servings: 3)

INGREDIENTS

- 2 tbsp of olive oil
- 1 Pinch of sea salt
- 1 Crushed, finely chopped garlic clove
- 1 Seeded and finely chopped red Chile
- 5 Oz of whole Shishita peppers
- 10 Ounces of jumbo shrimp
- 2 tbsp of low-sodium light soy sauce
- The juice of 1 lime

Directions:

1. Heat your Air Fryer to a temperature of about 180 C for about 5 minutes
2. Spray your Air Fryer pan with olive oil
3. Add in the salt; the garlic and the red Chile and mix your ingredients very well
4. Add in the shishita peppers and mix; then add the shrimp and drizzle with a little bit of sesame oil
5. Place the baking pan in your Air Fryer and lock the lid
6. Set the timer to about 10 minutes and set the temperature to about 200° C/ 400°F

7. When the timer beeps; turn off your Air Fryer; and remove the pan
8. Transfer your ingredients to a serving bowl
9. Season your shrimp and peppers with the lime juice and the soy sauce
10. Serve and enjoy your delicious dish!

Nutrition facts

Amount per Serving

Calories- 101 g.

Fats- 8 g.

Fibre- 3.2 g.

Carbohydrate- 3 g.

Protein- 18 g.

The nutritional details are in general estimate and they should only be used like a guide with approximate use

Recipe 25: Stuffed Chicken

(Prep time: 8 minutes\ Cook Time: 25 minutes\ Servings: 4)

INGREDIENTS:

- 4 Chicken breasts, Medium
- 1 tsp paprika
- 1 tsp salt, divided
- 1 ½ TBSP olive oil
- ¼ TBSP garlic powder
- ¼ tsp onion powder
- 2 TBSP mayonnaise
- 1 ¼ Cups fresh parsley, finely chopped
- ½ Cup black olive, hulled and sliced
- 1 tsp garlic, finely minced
- ½ tsp red pepper flakes

Directions:

1. Preheat the oven to about 375° degrees F
2. Arrange the chicken breasts over a cutting board; then drizzle it with olive oil
3. Add ½ teaspoon of the paprika, the salt, onion powder and garlic powder in a medium bowl and combine
4. Sprinkle the spices on both sides of the chicken breasts
5. Make a pocket on one side of each of the chicken breasts; then set the chicken aside

6. Add the mayonnaise, garlic, red pepper, the olive, 1 pinch of salt and the parsley and mix; then spoon the mixture evenly into each of the chicken breasts
7. Arrange the stuffed chicken breasts in a 9x13 baking tray and bake for about 26 minutes
8. When the chicken is perfectly cooked, remove from the oven
9. Serve and enjoy your delicious dish!

Nutrition facts
Amount per Serving
Calories-255 g.
Fats- 10.7 g.
Fibre- 0.3 g.
Carbohydrate-1.6 g.
Protein- 35 g.
The nutritional details are in general estimate and they should only be used like a guide with approximate use

Recipe 26: Beef Liver Skillet with Green Pepper

(Prep time: 5minutes\Cook Time: 15 minutes\ Servings: 3)

INGREDIENTS:

- 3 Medium green peppers, finely sliced into rounds
- 1 Pinch sea salt
- 1 Pinch ground black pepper, coarsely ground
- 3 Medium onions; peeled and finely sliced
- 3 Cloves garlic, finely minced
- 1lb Beef livers, chopped into cubes
- 1 ½ TBSP balsamic vinegar
- 3 Sprigs fresh parsley, organic and finely chopped

Directions:

1. Add the garlic, chopped pepper and onions into a large and heavy skillet and over medium high heat
2. Season with black pepper and salt and stir for about 12 minutes
3. Add the beef livers and season it with 1 pinch of salt and cook for 3 minutes
4. Toss your ingredients very well; then drizzle with the balsamic vinegar and cook for about 1 additional minute

5. Remove the skillet from the heat and top with chopped fresh parsley
6. Serve and enjoy your gorgeous dish!

Nutrition facts

Amount per Serving

Calories- 261 g.

Fats- 12 g.

Fibre- 0.1 g.

Carbohydrate- 7 g.

Protein- 28 g.

The nutritional details are in general estimate and they should only be used like a guide with approximate use

Recipe 27: Beef and Sweet Potato Skillet

(Prep time: 8 minutes\ Cook Time: 27 minutes\ Servings: 4)

INGREDIENTS:

For the Beef preparation:

- 1 ¼ lbs beef, ground
- 1 Medium onion, finely diced
- 1 Medium green bell pepper, finely diced
- 1 clove garlic, minced
- 1 tsp paprika
- 1 tsp cumin, ground
- 1 ¼ tsp Chilli powder
- 1 tsp oregano, dried
- 2 TBSP coconut oil, melted
- 2 Medium green onions, sliced
- 1 Pinch sea salt
- 1 Pinch black pepper, freshly ground

For the sweet potatoes:

- 2 Large sweet potatoes, peeled and finely diced
- ½ Juice lime
- 2 TBSP olive oil, extra virgin
- 1 ½ tsp chilli powder
- ¼ tsp cumin
- 1 Pinch salt
- 1 pinch black pepper; freshly ground

Directions:

1. Preheat an oven to 425° F.
2. In a large bowl; combine the lime juice, olive oil, chilli powder, lime juice, cumin, pepper and salt
3. Toss the potatoes into the mixture and coat well; then transfer the potatoes to a baking sheet
4. Place the baking sheet in the oven and roast the potatoes for 18 to 20 minutes
5. Melt the coconut oil in a large skillet over medium high heat and add in the onion; then sauté for about 2 minutes
6. Add the garlic and sauté for about 1 additional minute
7. Add in the ground beef and cook for about 7 minutes; then add in the bell pepper and cook for about 3 minutes
8. Add the cumin, chilli powder, oregano and paprika, and season with 1 pinch salt and pepper
9. Garnish with finely chopped green onions
10. Serve the cooked ground beef with the sweet potatoes and enjoy!

Nutrition facts
Amount per Serving
Calories- 276 g.
Fats- 13.6 g.
Fibre- 1.1 g.
Carbohydrate- 9.6 g.
Protein- 18 g.

The nutritional details are in general estimate and they should only be used like a guide with approximate use

Recipe 28: Stuffed Pork

(Prep time: 6 minutes\ Cook Time: 50 minutes\ Servings: 5)

INGREDIENTS:

- 2 ½ lbs pork tenderloin
- 1 Medium red onion, finely chopped
- 3 Oz mushrooms, finely chopped
- 1 tsp coconut oil, melted
- 1 Large apple, peeled and finely chopped
- 1 Medium lemon, zest
- 1 Pinch salt
- 1 Pinch black pepper
- 2 TBSP olive oil
- ¼ tsp nutmeg
- 1 Bay leaf
- 1 Cup water

Directions:

1. Preheat an oven to about 350 degrees Fahrenheit
2. Melt the coconut oil in a medium pot over medium high heat; then add in the onion, apple and mushroom and sauté for about 2 to 3 minutes
3. Season with salt, nutmeg, lemon zest and pepper and stir

4. Remove from the pan from the heat and set it aside; then soak 6 toothpicks into cold water
5. Rinse the pork meat and pat it dry with paper towels
6. With a kitchen knife, make an incision down the length of the pork tenderloin; but don't cut it all the way through
7. Open the meat just the way you open a book; then cover with a plastic wrap and pound with the flat side of a meat mallet
8. Cover the pork meat with a plastic wrap and pound until the meat gets ½ inch thickness
9. Spread the mushroom and apple mixture on top of the pork meat and start rolling
10. Tightly roll the tenderloin; then secure all the seams with the rinsed and soaked toothpicks
11. Brush the pork roll with the olive oil and season with 1 pinch of salt and 1 pinch of pepper
12. Preheat a large; heavy frying pan and spray it with olive oil; then place the pork tenderloin in the bottom of the pan
13. Sauté the pork roll for about 5 minutes: then transfer it to a baking tray and bake for about 45 minutes at 375° F
14. Remove the pork roll from the oven and let rest for about 4 minutes
15. Slice the meat roll; then serve and enjoy it with chopped avocado!

Nutrition facts
Amount per Serving
Calories- 130 g.

Fats- 11.4 g.
Fibre- 0.8 g.
Carbohydrate- 0.1 g.
Protein- 6.7 g.

The nutritional details are in general estimate and they should only be used like a guide with approximate use

Recipe 29: Baked Talipa with Lemon and Mushrooms

(Prep time: 7 minutes\ Cook Time: 15 minutes\ Servings: 4-5)

INGREDIENTS:

- ¼ Cup coconut oil, melted
- 2 TBSP lemon juice, freshly squeezed
- 4 cloves garlic, finely minced
- 1 lemon, zest
- 4 tilapia fillets, about 6 Oz
- 1 Pinch salt
- 1 Pinch black pepper, freshly ground
- 2 TBSP fresh parsley, finely chopped

Directions:
1. Preheat an oven to about 425° Fahrenheit
2. Lightly spray 9x13 baking tray with cooking spray
3. In a medium bowl, combine the garlic, melted coconut oil, lemon zest and lemon juice and set aside
4. Season the tilapia with pepper and salt: then place it in the baking tray and drizzle with the prepared lemon mixture
5. Place the tray in the oven and bake for about 10 to 12 minutes
6. Remove the tray from the oven and garnish with parsley

7. Serve and enjoy your dish!

Nutrition facts

Amount per Serving

Calories- 174.5 g.

Fats- 7.4 g.

Fibre- 0.3 g.

Carbohydrate- 2.2 g.

Protein- 26 g.

The nutritional details are in general estimate and they should only be used like a guide with approximate use

Recipe 30: Salmon with Orange Sauce

(Prep time: 10 minutes\ Cook Time: 10 minutes\ Servings: 3)

INGREDIENTS:

INGREDIENTS FOR THE SALMON:

- 1 lb salmon fillet
- 2 tsp ghee
- 1 tsp ginger, ground
- 1 Pinch salt
- 1 pinch black pepper, freshly ground

For the orange sauce:

- 1 TBSP lemon, Juice
- 3 Tbsp orange juice
- 1 Tbsp coconut oil, melted

Directions:

1. Melt the coconut oil in a heavy cast iron skillet over medium high heat
2. Sprinkle the salmon with ginger, sea salt and paprika
3. Make the orange sauce by stirring the juiced lemon with the orange juice and the melted coconut oil in a jar and shake the mixture
4. Place the salmon in the skillet and with the skin side down and cook for about 4 minutes

5. Lower the heat and flip the salmon to cook for about 4 minutes
6. Remove the salmon from the skillet and let rest for 2 minutes
7. Place the cooked salmon on a serving platter and serve it with the orange sauce
8. Enjoy your lunch!

Nutrition facts

Amount per Serving

Calories- 270 g.

Fats- 12.3 g.

Fibre- 1.2 g.

Carbohydrate- 5.5 g.

Protein- 32 g.

The nutritional details are in general estimate and they should only be used like a guide with approximate use

CHAPTER 9: KETOGENIC DIET SNACKS AND SIDES

Recipe 31: Beet Salad

(Prep time: 5 minutes\ Cook Time: 5 minutes\ Servings: 3)

INGREDIENTS:

- 2 Large beets, peeled, boiled and chopped
- 1 Small white onion, peeled and chopped
- 1 Medium ripe tomato, finely chopped
- 2 TBSP olive oil
- 2 TBSP Chives and parsley, fresh and finely chopped
- 3 TBSP olive oil
- 2 TBSP balsamic vinegar
- 1 Pinch salt
- 1 Pinch black pepper, freshly ground

Directions:

1. Combine the diced avocado, onion, tomato and beets in a large mixing bowl
2. In a separate shallow dish, mix the vinegar with the oil, salt, herbs and pepper
3. Dress your veggies with the vinegar and oil and toss very well
4. Refrigerate the salad for about 1 hour
5. Garnish with chopped chives and flat parsley

6. Serve and enjoy your salad!

Nutrition facts
Amount per Serving
Calories- 93 g.
Fats- 4.2 g.
Fibre- 0.3 g.
Carbohydrate- 2.1 g.
Protein- 6.7 g.

The nutritional details are in general estimate and they should only be used like a guide with approximate use

Recipe 32: Sweet Potato Fritters

(Prep time: 5 minutes\ Cook Time: 20 minutes\ Servings: 5-6)

INGREDIENTS:

- 1 Medium sweet potato
- 2 Medium white onions, finely chopped
- 1 Cup parsley, finely chopped
- 2 Cups fresh dill, finely chopped
- 1 Cup chicken liver
- 1 tsp red pepper
- 1 Pinch black pepper
- 1 Pinch salt
- 1 Pinch mint, dry
- 2 Large eggs
- 3 TBSP Olive oil

Directions:

1. Place a medium pan filled with water over medium high heat and bring it to a boil
2. Toss in the sweet potato and cook for about 10 to 12 minutes
3. Remove the potato from the pan and peel it
4. Cook the chicken liver after rinsing it with water
5. Mash the potato with a potato masher in a medium bowl and add to it the chicken liver and mash again

6. Add in the chopped white onion, the chopped parsley and dill
7. Season the mixture with the red pepper, the black pepper, the mint and the salt and mix very well
8. Add the egg and mix very well
9. Heat the olive oil in a large skillet over medium high heat and let it heat for 1 and ½ minutes
10. Make small fritters of the sweet potato and dill mixture and fry it in the skillet for about 3 minutes; then flip the fritters and cook for about 4 minutes
11. Remove the fritters and let cool for 2 minutes
12. Serve and enjoy your fritters!

Nutrition facts
Amount per Serving
Calories- 136 g.
Fats- 6.2 g.
Fibre- 0.7 g.
Carbohydrate- 3 g.
Protein- 8 g.
The nutritional details are in general estimate and they should only be used like a guide with approximate use

Recipe 33: Eggplant Fries

(Prep time: 3 minutes\ Cook Time: 20 minutes\ Servings: 3)

INGREDIENTS

- 1 Medium, sliced eggplant
- 2 Cups of almond meal
- 2 Teaspoons of fresh rosemary
- 1 and ½ teaspoons of dried thyme
- 1 Teaspoon of smoked paprika
- ¾ Teaspoon of salt
- 2 Large eggs
- 2 Tablespoons of extra virgin olive oil
- To make the dipping Sauce:
- ½ Cup of organic mayonnaise
- ¼ Teaspoon of chilli powder
- ¼ Teaspoon of smoked paprika
- ¼ Teaspoon of Dijon mustard

Directions

1. Preheat your oven to about 450° F
2. Line a baking sheet with a parchment paper
3. Stir the almond meal with the rosemary, the thyme, the paprika, and the salt into a large dish.
4. In another dish, mix the egg with the olive oil and dip the eggplant slices into the mixture of the egg
5. Dredge the eggplant slices in the almond flour

6. Place the eggplant slices over the baking sheet; then bake the eggplant fries in the oven for about 20 minutes
7. Serve and enjoy your fries!

Nutrition facts
Amount per Serving
Calories- 233.5 g.
Fats- 17.4 g.
Fibre- 0.8 g.
Carbohydrate- 8.4 g.
Protein- 11.6 g.

The nutritional details are in general estimate and they should only be used like a guide with approximate use

Recipe 34: Sweet Potato Mash

(Prep time: 15 minutes\ Cook Time: 30 minutes\ Servings: 5)

INGREDIENTS

- 5 large peeled and chopped sweet potatoes
- 3 Tablespoons of ghee
- 3 Tablespoons of maple syrup
- 1 Teaspoon of vanilla extract
- 2 Teaspoons of cinnamon
- 1 Pinch of nutmeg
- 1 Pinch of salt
- 1 Cup of chopped walnuts
- ½ Cup of unsweetened chopped coconut flakes
- 2 Tablespoons of coconut oil

Directions:

1. Fill a large pot with water and let boil for about 12 minutes
2. Toss the potatoes into the boiling water and let simmer for about 10 minutes
3. Remove the potatoes from the heat and let it drain
4. Preheat your oven to about 350° F.
5. Add about 2 tablespoons of maple syrup and ghee to the sweet potatoes; then add the vanilla, 1 teaspoon of cinnamon, the nutmeg and the salt

6. Mash your potatoes with the rest of the ingredients
7. Season with the salt and transfer the mashed potatoes to a serving platter
8. In a separate bowl; mix the coconut flakes with the walnuts, the coconut oil, the ghee and the syrup; then sprinkle with cinnamon
9. Top the sweet potatoes with walnuts and bake it for about 19 minutes
10. Serve and enjoy!

Nutrition facts
Amount per Serving
Calories- 151.1 g.
Fats- 3.7 g.
Fibre- 0.2g.
Carbohydrate- 18 g.
Protein- 5 g.
The nutritional details are in general estimate and they should only be used like a guide with approximate use

Recipe 35: Cauliflower Sticks

(Prep time: 4 minutes\ Cook Time: 29 minutes\ Servings: 7)

INGREDIENTS

- 1 Medium cauliflower head
- ½ Tablespoon of oregano
- 1 Tablespoon of basil
- 1 Tablespoon of onion powder
- ½ Teaspoon of red pepper flakes
- 2 Large eggs
- 1 Pinch of salt and pepper

Directions

1. Microwave the entire head of cauliflower in a heat proof dish for about 10 minutes
2. Remove the cauliflower from the microwave and pulse it in a food processor until it becomes smooth
3. Refrigerate the cauliflower for about 10 minutes; then combine the remaining ingredients with it
4. Prepare a baking sheet by greasing it with a little bit of oil
5. Press down the cauliflower into the baking sheet until it becomes of about ½ inch of thickness
6. Put the baking sheet in the oven for about 24 minutes and the heat to about 425° F

7. Remove the cauliflower from the oven and set it to a broil at about 500
8. Cut the cauliflower into sticks; then flip it and put it back in the oven and cook it for about 15 minutes
9. Serve and enjoy!

Nutrition facts
Amount per Serving
Calories- 163 g.
Fats- 9.8 g.
Fibre- 0.5 g.
Carbohydrate- 4.5 g.
Protein- 5.1 g.

The nutritional details are in general estimate and they should only be used like a guide with approximate use

Recipe 36: Southern-Style Salad

(Prep time: 5 minutes\ Cook Time: 35 minutes\ Servings: 4)

INGREDIENTS

- 2 Pounds of sweet potatoes
- 1 Pinch of sea salt
- 4 Large beaten eggs
- 1/3 Cup of Pistachios
- 1 and ¼ cups of diced cucumber
- 1 Cup of cubed Roma Tomato
- ½ Cup of roughly chopped Cilantro
- ½ Cup of thinly sliced Dates
- 3 Tablespoons of thinly sliced fresh mint
- Components to prepare the dressing:
- 1 Cup of roasted soaked cashews
- 7 and ½ tablespoons of Water
- 2 Tablespoons and 1 teaspoon of fresh lemon juice
- 1 Tablespoon of Lemon zest
- 2 and ¼ teaspoons of ground cumin
- 2 and ¼ teaspoon of fresh minced ginger
- 1 and ½ teaspoons of ground cinnamon
- 1 Teaspoon of sea salt
- ¼ Teaspoon of Paprika
- ¼ Teaspoon of Ground allspice
- 1 Pinch of pepper

Directions:

1. Rinse and cut the potatoes into small cubes; then put it in a large saucepan and sprinkle with salt
2. Let your ingredients boil over a medium heat and cook for about 20 minutes
3. Drain the potatoes and set it aside to cool
4. Put the eggs into a medium pan and cover it with water; then boil it for about 10 minutes
5. Set the eggs aside to cool; then preheat the oven to about 375° F and toast the pistachios until it becomes golden for about 10 minutes
6. Drain the water from the cashews and put it in a blender
7. Add the rest of the dressing elements and blend all together until your ingredients become smooth
8. Peel the skin of the boiled potatoes; then chop it into cubes of ¾ inch each
9. Add the cucumber, the tomato, the cilantro, the dates, the mint and the chopped pistachios.
10. Peel your eggs and chop it; then add it to the bowl and pour your prepared dressing on top of the salad

Nutrition facts
Amount per Serving
Calories- 152 g.
Fats- 3.7 g.
Fibre- 0.2 g.
Carbohydrate- 18 g.
Protein- 5 g.
The nutritional details are in general estimate and they should only be used like a guide with approximate use

Recipe 37: Onion Fries

(Prep time: 3 minutes\ Cook Time: 5 minutes\ Servings: 2)

INGREDIENTS

- 1 Onion
- ½ Cup of coconut flour
- ¼ Cup of arrowroot powder
- ½ Teaspoon of garlic powder
- 1 Teaspoon of salt
- ½ Teaspoon of pepper
- 2 Large eggs
- Coconut oil

Directions:

1. Heat the coconut oil over medium high heat in a large non-stick skillet
2. Mix the coconut flour, the arrowroot and the spices over a large dish
3. Beat the eggs in a large bowl
4. Peel; then thinly slice a whole onion into thin rings
5. Separate the rings, then dip it into the egg mixture and later in the mixture of the coconut
6. Drop the onion rings in the heated oil; then cook it for about 2 to 3 minutes per side
7. Remove the onion and set it aside to cool
8. Serve and enjoy your onion rings!

Nutrition facts
Amount per Serving
Calories- 141 g.
Fats- 10 g.
Fibre- 2.1 g.
Carbohydrate- 9 g.
Protein- 7.2 g.

The nutritional details are in general estimate and they should only be used like a guide with approximate use

Recipe 38: Fried Spinach with Cashew Cream

(Prep time: 7 minutes\ Cook Time: 11 minutes\ Servings: 3)

INGREDIENTS:

- 2 Boxes of 10 Oz each chopped spinach
- 2 Cans of 14 Oz of artichoke hearts
- 1 Tablespoon of extra-virgin olive oil
- 1 Small diced onion
- 2 Minced garlic cloves
- 1 and ½ teaspoons of sea salt
- 1 Teaspoon of onion powder
- ½ Teaspoon of garlic powder
- ½ Teaspoon of black pepper
- ¼ Teaspoon of cayenne pepper
- 1 Tablespoon of lemon juice
- 1 and ½ cups of cashew cream

Directions:

1. Start by defrosting the spinach; then squeeze out any excess of water; then set it aside
2. Drain; then cut the artichokes
3. Pour the olive oil in a pan; then sauté for about 10 minutes with the onion
4. Add the garlic; then cook for about 1 minute
5. Add the artichoke; the salt, the onion powder, the garlic powder, the black pepper and the cayenne; then heat your ingredients.

6. Add the spinach and the lemon juice; then stir very well
7. Add the cashew cream
8. Serve and enjoy!

Nutrition facts

Amount per Serving

Calories- 116 g.

Fats- 3 g.

Fibre- 0.4 g.

Carbohydrate- 12 g.

Protein- 13.5 g.

The nutritional details are in general estimate and they should only be used like a guide with approximate use

Recipe 39: Stir-Fried Garlicky Mushrooms

(Prep time: 5 minutes\ Cook Time: 15minutes\ Servings: 4-5)

INGREDIENTS:

- 1 Pound of white button mushrooms
- 3 Tablespoons of bacon fat
- 1 Small, finely chopped white onion
- 2 Chopped garlic cloves garlic
- ½ Teaspoon of sea salt
- ¼ Teaspoon of ground black pepper
- 1 and ½ tablespoons of balsamic vinegar
- 1 Tablespoon of chopped fresh parsley

Directions:

1. Start by cleaning and wiping your mushrooms gently with a damp paper; then slice each one in halves and set it aside
2. Put the bacon fat in a large non-stick skillet over a medium heat
3. Add in the mushrooms, the onion and the garlic; then cook for about 9 minutes
4. Cook the mushrooms until it becomes tender and stir through the process
5. Season with the sea salt, the pepper and the balsamic vinegar; then stir very well to combine your ingredients.
6. Cook for about 2 minutes; then garnish with parsley

7. Serve and enjoy!

Nutrition facts

Amount per Serving

Calories- 193 g.

Fats- 13.7 g.

Fibre- 0.3 g.

Carbohydrate- 4 g.

Protein- 13.7 g.

The nutritional details are in general estimate and they should only be used like a guide with approximate use

Recipe 40: Gluten-Free Tortillas

(Prep time: 15 minutes\ Cook Time: 20 minutes\ Servings: 3)

INGREDIENTS:

- 1 Cup almond flour, blanched
- 1 Cup Arrowroot Flour
- 1 Pinch Sea Salt
- ½ tsp baking powder, grain free
- 2 Large eggs
- 1 Cup coconut milk
- ¼ TBSP coconut oil

Directions:

1. Whisk all together the arrowroot flour, almond flour, baking powder and salt in a large mixing bowl
2. Crack the eggs in a bowl and gradually add in the milk; then combine until the mixture is very well mixed
3. Pour the egg and coconut milk mixture into the bowl with the dry ingredients
4. Combine the ingredients very well and if it is too thick; you can add 1 additional tablespoon of coconut milk and if you want the mixture to be smooth, blend it with a blender
5. Place a large non-stick skillet over medium high heat and spray it with the coconut oil

6. When the coconut oil is melted, pour about 1/3 to ½ cup of the batter into the skillet and the way to do it is easy; just lift the cup and swirl it, pour it in the pan and swirl to spread the batter
7. Let cook for about 1 to 2 minutes or until the bottoms starting getting firm
8. Flip the tortilla and cook for about 2 additional minutes; then remove it and set it aside
9. Repeat the same process with the remaining quantity of batter; you will have about 6 tortillas by the end
10. Serve and enjoy your tortillas!

Nutrition facts
Amount per Serving
Calories- 177 g.
Fats- 9 g.
Fibre- 1.7 g.
Carbohydrate- 11.2 g.
Protein- 6.8 g.

The nutritional details are in general estimate and they should only be used like a guide with approximate use

CHAPTER 10: KETOGENIC DIET DINNER RECIPES

Recipe 41: Beef Picadillo

(Prep time: 10 minutes\ Cook Time: 20 minutes\ Servings: 4)

INGREDIENTS

- 2 Tablespoons of olive oil
- 3 Medium, finely chopped garlic cloves
- 1 Medium, finely chopped yellow onion finely
- 1 Medium, finely chopped red bell pepper
- 1 and ½ pounds of Ground beef
- 2 Teaspoons of kosher salt
- 1 Teaspoon of black pepper
- 1 Teaspoon of paprika
- 1 Teaspoon of dried oregano
- 1 Teaspoon of ground cumin
- 1 to 2 dried bay leaves
- 1 Cup of canned, non salted chopped tomatoes
- 1 Tablespoon of tomato paste
- ¼ Cup of chopped Pimento Stuffed olives
- 2 Tablespoons of olive brine
- 2 Tablespoons of water
- 1 Tablespoon of raisins
- 1 Handful of chopped fresh cilantro

Directions:

1. Peel; then chop the garlic or finely mince it with the onion
2. Remove the cores of the olives and deseed the bell pepper
3. Mix the spices into a small tray; then slice the olives, the raisins, the tomatoes and the tomato paste; then add the olive brine and the water
4. Heat a skillet over a medium heat and once your ingredients become hot, add the olive oil with the garlic, the onion and the bell pepper
5. Sauté your ingredients for about 7 minutes and keep stirring until your onions become translucent.
6. Add in the Ground beef and after that raise the heat to medium
7. With a wooden spatula; break the ground pieces of beef with a spatula
8. Toss in the salt, the pepper, the paprika, the oregano; the cumin and the bay leaf. Cook your ingredients and stir it until it is perfectly mixed
9. Add the diced tomatoes, the tomato paste, the sliced olives, the olive juice and the water
10. Add the raisins and toss very well to mix your ingredients; then let simmer for about 20 minutes
11. Stir in the chopped cilantro; then serve over the cauliflower rice
12. Enjoy your dinner!

Nutrition facts
Amount per Serving

Calories- 178.5 g.

Fats- 7.8 g.

Fibre- 1.7 g.

Carbohydrate- 7.7 g.

Protein- 20.4 g.

The nutritional details are in general estimate and they should only be used like a guide with approximate use

Recipe 42: Chicken Fajitas

(Prep time: 10 minutes\ Cook Time: 25 minutes\ Servings: 4-5)

INGREDIENTS

- 4 Butterflied chicken breasts
- 1 Sliced bell pepper
- 1 Sliced red onion
- The juice of 1 lime
- ¼ Cup of olive oil
- 1 Minced garlic clove
- 2 Tablespoon of fresh cilantro
- ½ Teaspoon of cumin
- 1 Teaspoon of chilli powder
- 1 Teaspoon of dried oregano
- ¼ Teaspoon of cayenne pepper
- 1 Pinch of sea salt
- 1 Pinch of freshly ground black pepper
- Fresh chopped cilantro

Directions:

1. Preheat the grill to a medium-high heat.
2. In a large bowl, combine altogether the lime juice, the olive oil, the garlic, the fresh cilantro, the cumin, the chilli powder, the oregano, and the cayenne pepper
3. Season the chicken with a little bit of salt and 1 pinch of pepper to taste.

4. Put half of the mixture of the spice in a medium bowl; then add the bell pepper and the onion.
5. Arrange the chicken and fill it with the onion, the bell pepper, and the mixture of the spice.
6. Now, roll the chicken meat tightly and secure it with toothpicks
7. Brush the chicken with the mixture of the spice
8. Grill your chicken meat over a medium-high heat for about 25 minutes and flip it every 5 minutes
9. Serve and enjoy your chicken fajitas

Nutrition facts
Amount per Serving
Calories- 258 g.
Fats- 8 g.
Fibre- 2 g.
Carbohydrate- 13 g.
Protein- 29 g.
The nutritional details are in general estimate and they should only be used like a guide with approximate use

Recipe 43: Teriyaki Burgers with Pineapple Salsa

(Prep time: 6 minutes\ Cook Time: 30 minutes\ Servings: 3)

INGREDIENTS:

For the burgers

- 2 lbs ground turkey, grass-fed
- ⅓ Cup pineapple juice, sugar-free
- 1 tablespoon extra virgin oil
- 2 ½ TBSP coconut aminos
- 1 tsp sesame seeds
- 3 Cloves garlic, finely minced
- ½ tsp ginger, finely grated
- ½ tsp salt
- ¼ tsp red pepper flakes
- 1 Pineapple, medium

For the salsa

- 1 Medium mango, peeled and finely chopped
- ½ Cup nightshade baby tomatoes
- 2 TBSP basil, chopped
- 2 TBSP pineapple juice
- 1 TSP ginger, finely grated
- 1 clove garlic, finely minced
- ¼ tsp sea salt

Directions:

1. Start by combining the pineapple juice with the olive oil, coconut aminos, sesame seeds,

red pepper flakes, garlic and ginger in a large bowl

2. Add the ground turkey to the mixture you have just prepared and knead pretty well; then cover and let refrigerate for about 30 minutes

3. Combine the peeled and finely chopped mango with the ½ cup of baby tomatoes; the chopped basil, the ginger, garlic, pineapple juice and salt and process all with a food processor until you obtain a roughly chopped mixture

4. Refrigerate the salsa for about 15 minutes

5. Peel the pineapple and slice it into rings; you would want to have about 5 pieces, so if there are any left, just store it in the refrigerator

6. Preheat your grill to medium high heat and make patties from the marinated meat with both your hands

7. Arrange the turkey patties directly on top of the grill and grill it for about 4 minutes per side

8. Remove the turkey patties from the grill and place it in a foil

9. Grill the pineapple rounds for about 1 minute per side; then remove it and get ready to assemble your burgers

10. Place each pineapple ring on top of the turkey patties

11. Serve your burgers on a bed of lettuce leaves and top it with the mango salsa; enjoy!

Nutrition facts

Amount per Serving

Calories- 219 g.
Fats- 6.7 g.
Fibre- 2.3 g.
Carbohydrate- 10.9 g.
Protein- 22 g.

The nutritional details are in general estimate and they should only be used like a guide with approximate use

Recipe 44: Spaghetti Squash

(Prep time: 8 minutes\ Cook Time: 50 minutes\ Servings: 4)

INGREDIENTS

- 2 and ½ pounds of medium spaghetti squash
- 4 Tablespoons of coconut oil
- 2 Minced garlic cloves
- 1 Diced medium carrot
- 2 Diced stalks of celery
- ½ Minced medium yellow onion
- 1 Small, diced red bell pepper
- 1 Pound of ground chicken
- 1 Teaspoon of garlic powder
- 1 Teaspoon of fine sea salt
- ¼ Teaspoon of black pepper
- 1 Cup of hot sauce
- ¼ Cup of Super Simple
- 3 Large eggs, chopped and whisked chopped scallions
- 1 Sliced avocado

Directions:

1. Preheat your oven to about 390°F.
2. Cut the spaghetti squash into two halves; then place the squash on top of a baking sheet
3. Bake the squash spaghetti for about 30 minutes

4. Remove the squash from the oven; then lower the temperature to about 350°F.
5. Grease a medium baking tray with cooking spray and remove its threads
6. Set the squash aside to cool for a few minutes
7. Transfer the squash threads to a greased baking tray
8. In a large skillet and over a medium heat, melt about 2 tablespoons of coconut oil.
9. Add the carrots, the garlic, the celery, the onion, and the bell pepper; then cook for about 9 minutes
10. Add the garlic powder, the ground chicken, the salt, and the pepper; then cook for a few minutes; about 7 minutes
11. Remove the skillet from the heat and add the sauce and the mayonnaise; then stir very well
12. Pour the mixture of the chicken and add to it the spaghetti squash threads in a baking tray.
13. Add the eggs and mix very well
14. Bake the tray in the oven for about 55 minutes
15. Garnish the tray with the chopped scallion and with avocado slices.
16. Serve and enjoy!

Nutrition facts
Amount per Serving
Calories- 228 g.
Fats- 8.1 g.
Fibre- 1 g.
Carbohydrate- 15 g.
Protein- 13.8 g.
The nutritional details are in general estimate and they should only be used like a guide with approximate use

Recipe 45: Beef Roll

(Prep time: 7 minutes\ Cook Time: 20 minutes\ Servings: 6-7)

INGREDIENTS:

- 2 lbs steak, flank
- 2 Small onions, sweet and finely chopped
- 2 TBSP olive oil, divided
- 2 ½ TBSP garlic, finely chopped
- 2 ¼ Cups mushrooms, thinly sliced
- ½ TBSP kosher salt
- 1 Pinch black pepper, freshly ground
- 1 Cup baby spinach, fresh and finely chopped

Directions:

1. Preheat an oven to about 375° Fahrenheit.
2. In a large pan and over medium high heat, pour 1 tablespoon of the oil and heat it; then add in the onions, mushrooms, salt, garlic and pepper and cook for about 15 minutes
3. Remove the pan from the heat and set it aside; then place the flank steak over a cutting board
4. Spoon the onion and mushroom mixture and evenly spread it
5. Sprinkle the baby spinach on top; then press down with your hands and start rolling tightly

6. Secure the steak roll with 6 toothpicks in the centre and sides; make sure that nothing of the stuffing is outside the beef roll
7. Spray a large skillet with a tablespoon of olive oil and let heat for 1 minute; then sear the steak roll for about 2 minutes per side
8. Transfer the skillet to the oven and bake for about 12 to 15 minutes
9. Remove the toothpicks; then slice the beef roll
10. Serve and enjoy your meal!

Nutrition facts
Amount per Serving
Calories- 275 g.
Fats- 11 g.
Fibre- 1 g.
Carbohydrate- 8.9 g.
Protein- 29 g.
The nutritional details are in general estimate and they should only be used like a guide with approximate use

Recipe 46: Beef Meatballs with Sweet Potato Mash

(Prep time: 10 minutes\ Cook Time: 15 minutes\ Servings: 6)

INGREDIENTS

- 1 and ½ pounds of ground beef;
- 1 large egg
- 2 Tablespoons of old fashioned mustard
- 1 Tablespoon of coconut aminos;
- 1 Teaspoon of onion powder
- Coconut oil
- Minced fresh parsley
- 1 Pinch of Sea salt
- 1 Pinch of ground black pepper
- Ingredients to make the gravy
- 1 Chopped onion
- 1 Cup of beef stock
- 2 Tablespoons of clarified coconut oil
- 1 Pinch of Sea salt and 1 pinch of freshly ground black pepper

Ingredients to make the mashed potatoes:

- 4 Large peeled and chopped sweet potatoes
- 3 Tablespoons of clarified butter
- 1 Pinch of sea salt and 1 pinch of freshly ground black pepper

Directions:

1. Start by cooking the potatoes and boil it in hot water for about 14 to 15 minutes
2. After draining the potatoes; mash it with a potato masher and add the coconut oil; then season it with 1 pinch of black pepper and 1 pinch of salt
3. In a medium deep bowl, mix the ground beef, the egg; the mustard, the coconut aminos and the onion powder; then season your ingredients with a little bit of salt and with 1 pinch of ground black pepper
4. Shape your meat mixture into the form of meatballs with both your hands.
5. Melt a little bit of coconut oil into a large skillet over a medium heat
6. Toss the meatballs into the skillet; then cook it for a few minutes
7. Remove your meatballs from the skillet and set it aside
8. Without removing the skillet off the heat, add a little bit of coconut oil; then toss in the onion and sauté for a few minutes
9. Pour in the beef stock and return your meatballs to the same skillet; then gently add the gravy
10. Serve your meatballs with the seasoned and mashed potatoes; then top with fresh parsley
11. Serve and enjoy your dinner!

Nutrition facts
Amount per Serving

Calories- 271 g.
Fats- 11.8 g.
Fibre- 0.8 g.
Carbohydrate- 112 g.
Protein- 27 g.

The nutritional details are in general estimate and they
should only be used like a guide with approximate use

Recipe 47: Glazed Meatloaf

(Prep time: 5 minutes\ Cook Time: 60 minutes\ Servings: 5)

INGREDIENTS

- 2 Pounds of grass-fed ground beef
- 1 Large diced onion
- 1 Cup of cooked sweet potato
- 1 Cup of almond flour
- 2 Tablespoons of coconut flour
- 1 Large egg
- 1 Cup of gluten-free ketchup
- 3 Tablespoons of coconut aminos
- 2 Teaspoons of salt
- 1 Teaspoon of garlic powder

For the glaze

- ½ Cup of gluten free ketchup
- 2 Tablespoons of coconut aminos
- 1 Tablespoon of honey

Directions:

1. Preheat your oven to about 350° and prepare a baking tray by lining it with a cookie sheet or a parchment paper
2. Put the diced onion with a little bit of coconut oil in a saucepan; then sauté it until it becomes soft for about 6 minutes

3. In a large and deep bowl; mix altogether the beef, the onion, the sweet potato, the almond flour, the coconut flour, the egg, the ketchup, the coconut aminos, the salt, and the garlic powder together.
4. Make the form of a loaf and put it into a pan; then mix all the ingredients of the glaze in a bowl and pour it over the meatloaf
5. Bake your meatloaf for about 60 minutes; then remove it from the oven.
6. Set the meatloaf aside to cool; then slice it, serve and enjoy it!

Nutrition facts
Amount per Serving
Calories- 284 g.
Fats- 14 g.
Fibre- 1 g.
Carbohydrate- 10.6 g.
Protein- 29.6 g.
The nutritional details are in general estimate and they should only be used like a guide with approximate use

Recipe 48: Bacon Stuffed Beef Mignon

(Prep time: 9 minutes\ Cook Time: 15 minutes\ Servings: 4-5)

INGREDIENTS

- 2 Beef filet mignon
- 4 to 5 Pieces of bacon
- ⅛ Teaspoon of garlic powder
- 1 Pinch of salt
- 1 Pinch of black pepper
- 2 Tablespoons of mustard
- 1 Tablespoon of raw honey
- 1 Tablespoon of orange juice

Directions:

1. Preheat your oven to about 375 degrees.
2. Wrap each of the beef filet mignon with the pieces of the bacon so that you cover all the parts of the sides of the beef filet mignon.
3. Secure the filets of the beef mignon with the help of toothpicks and sprinkle a little bit of garlic powder, a little bit of salt and 1 pinch of black pepper
4. Put a large saucepan over medium high heat; then put each of the filets mignon and sauté it until it is perfectly cooked
5. Sear both of the tops and the bottoms of the fillets for about 3 minutes over each side

6. Transfer the mignon to the oven and add to it the mustard, the honey and the orange juice
7. Once cooked, serve and enjoy your dish!

Nutrition facts

Amount per Serving

Calories- 246 g.

Fats- 11 g.

Fibre- 1 g.

Carbohydrate- 3 g.

Protein- 35 g.

The nutritional details are in general estimate and they should only be used like a guide with approximate use

Recipe 49: Tuna Salad

(Prep time: 4 minutes\ Cook Time: 5 minutes\ Servings: 2)

INGREDIENTS

- 1 Can of white drained Albacore Tuna
- ½ Large, diced red bell pepper
- ½ Peeled and cut large carrot
- ¼ Cup of diced grape tomatoes
- 1 Thinly sliced scallion; only use the green part
- 1 Small mashed avocado
- 1 Tablespoon of lemon juice
- ½ Teaspoon of fine grain sea salt

Directions:

1. In a large bowl, mix the diced veggies, the tuna, the mashed avocado, the lime juice, the sliced scallions, and the salt altogether until your ingredients are very well combined.
2. Serve your tuna salad with a wrap
3. Enjoy this delicious tuna salad or store it in the refrigerator and enjoy it later

Nutrition facts
Amount per Serving
Calories- 142 g.
Fats- 8 g.
Fibre- 0.9 g.

Carbohydrate- 5.4 g.
Protein- 12 g.

The nutritional details are in general estimate and they should only be used like a guide with approximate use

Recipe 50: Shrimp Salad

(Prep time: 5 minutes\ Cook Time: 5 minutes\ Servings: 3-4)

INGREDIENTS:

- 1 lb shrimp, frozen or fresh
- 1 TBSP extra virgin olive oil
- ½ Cup red or white onion, finely chopped
- 3 Roma tomatoes, finely diced
- 1 Medium jalapeno peppers, finely diced
- ½ avocado, diced
- 4 TBSP lime juice, fresh
- 1 handful cilantro, finely chopped
- 1 Pinch pepper
- 1 Pinch salt

Directions:

1. Place a large skillet over medium high heat and heat the extra virgin olive oil
2. Toss in the shrimp and sprinkle the pepper on top
3. Sauté the shrimp for about 3 to 5 minutes
4. Remove the shrimp from the skillet and chop into quite small pieces
5. Assemble your salad by placing the chopped tomatoes, jalapenos, chopped shrimp; cilantro and avocado in a large mixing bowl with the salt and stir
6. Pour the lime juice on top and give a final stir

7. Serve and enjoy your shrimp salad!

Nutrition facts

Amount per Serving

Calories- 168 g.

Fats- 4 g.

Fibre- 0.8 g.

Carbohydrate- 5.6 g.

Protein- 27.6 g.

The nutritional details are in general estimate and they should only be used like a guide with approximate use

CHAPTER 11: KETOGENIC DIET DESSERT RECIPES

Recipe 51: Almond Cookies

(Prep time: 5 minutes\ Cook Time: 20 minutes\ Servings: 8)

INGREDIENTS:

- 1/3 Cup Maple syrup
- 2 ½ Cups Almond Meal
- 1 ½ TBSP coconut oil, melted
- ½ tsp Vanilla Extract
- ½ tsp baking soda
- 1 Pinch salt
- 1 TBSP Water

Directions:

1. Preheat the oven to about 350 degrees F.
2. Combine the almond meal, the baking soda and the salt in a large mixing bowl and mix very well
3. In a separate bowl, mix the coconut oil with the maple syrup, the vanilla extract with 1 tablespoon of water and whisk until the mixture becomes smooth

4. Add the wet ingredients to the bowl with the dry ingredients and make sure you obtain a sticky and quite difficult to stir the batter
5. Line a baking sheet with a parchment paper and get ready to make the cookies and to fulfil that, shape the cookies into small balls of about 1" diameter each
6. Press down the dough balls a little bit with your hands; then arrange the cookies on top of the baking paper
7. Place the baking sheet in the oven and bake for about 9 to 10 minutes
8. Let the cookies rest for about 5 minutes
9. Serve and enjoy your gorgeous cookies!

Nutrition facts

Amount per Serving

Calories- 140 g.

Fats- 6 g.

Fibre- 1.3 g.

Carbohydrate- 11 g.

Protein- 27.6 g.

The nutritional details are in general estimate and they should only be used like a guide with approximate use

Recipe 52: Caramel Flan

(Prep time: 6 minutes\ Cook Time: 60 minutes\ Servings: 6)

INGREDIENTS

- 2 Cups coconut milk, full fat
- 6 Large pasteurized eggs, yolks
- ¼ Cup tapioca flour
- 3 TBSP honey, raw
- 1 TBSP vanilla, extract
- 1/3 Cup water, cool
- ½ Cup coconut sugar
- 2 TBSP shredded coconut, unsweetened

Directions:

1. Preheat an oven to about 350°F.
2. Make the caramel sauce by placing the coconut sugar with the water in a pan and bring the mixture to a simmer for about 5 to 6 minutes and stir from time to time
3. When the sauce starts to thicken; remove the pan from the heat and set it aside
4. Spoon about 2 tablespoons of the caramel sauce into the bottom of ramekins and let cool
5. Make the flan by placing the coconut milk, the egg yolks, the tapioca flour, the honey, the vanilla extract and the shredded coconut in a

food processor and process on high speed for about 30 seconds

6. Check the caramel to see if it has thickened; then pour the batter into the ramekins you have prepared

7. Put the ramekins in a deep baking tray and fill it with boiling water

8. Cover the ramekins with a foil and bake it in the oven for about 55 to 60 minutes

9. Remove the ramekins from the oven and let cool for about 20 minutes

10. Refrigerate the ramekins for about 4 hours

11. Top with the caramel sauce and shredded coconut; then serve and enjoy your flan

Nutrition facts

Amount per Serving

Calories- 265g.

Fats- 11.6 g.

Fibre- 0.4 g.

Carbohydrate- 13 g.

Protein- 7 g.

The nutritional details are in general estimate and they should only be used like a guide with approximate use

Recipe 53: Chocolate Chia Cookies

(Prep time: 8 minutes\ Cook Time: 30 minutes\ Servings: 10)

INGREDIENTS

- 2 tablespoons of organic Yacon syrup
- 1 vanilla extract
- 6 tablespoons of coconut milk
- 1 tablespoon of coconut oil
- 1 Cup of black chocolate (crushed)
- 1 Cup of organic chia flour
- 2 tablespoons of organic Maca
- 1/2 g yeast
- 1/2 g cinnamon
- 1 pinch of salt

Directions:

1. Mix well in a large bowl the Yacon syrup, the vanilla extract. Add coconut milk and coconut oil.
2. Mix the chia flour, Maca powder, yeast, cinnamon and salt in a small bowl and add to the previous mixture. Stir in the little pieces of chocolate.
3. Cover a plate with baking paper and place small balls of dough (about the size of a tablespoon).
4. Bake at 200 ° C/400° F for about 30 minutes.
5. The cookies are also delicious with white chocolate.

Nutrition facts

Amount per Serving

Calories- 73g.

Fats- 5 g.

Fibre- 1.7 g.

Carbohydrate- 3.9 g.

Protein- 4 g.

The nutritional details are in general estimate and they should only be used like a guide with approximate use

Recipe 54: Sesame Crackers

(Prep time: 7 minutes\ Cook Time: 20 minutes\ Servings: 7-8)

INGREDIENTS:

- ½ Cup of almond meal
- 1/3 Cup of sesame seeds
- 1 Teaspoon of olive oil
- 1 Large egg white
- 1 Pinch of salt
- 1 Pinch of pepper

Directions:

1. Preheat your oven to about 365° F.
2. Put all the ingredients into a large bowl and mix very well
3. Put the mixture over a baking sheet; then cover it with another baking sheet
4. Roll the mixture with a rolling pin
5. Score the pastry with the back of your knife into pieces shaped into squares
6. Remove the baking paper from the top of your pastry and transfer it to a baking pan
7. Put the pastry in the oven for about 18 minutes
8. Serve and enjoy!

Nutrition facts
Amount per Serving

Calories- 196 g.
Fats- 16 g.
Fibre- 0.5 g.
Carbohydrate- 6 g.
Protein- 8 g.

The nutritional details are in general estimate and they should only be used like a guide with approximate use

Recipe 55: Cocoa Truffles

(Prep time: 10 minutes\ Cook Time: 5 minutes\ Servings: 10)

INGREDIENTS

- 2 tablespoons of raw cocoa
- 3 tablespoons of flaxseed oatmeal
- 2 cups of peanut butter/or chia butter
- 1 tablespoon of organic chia seeds
- 2 tablespoons of Protein powder

Directions:

1. Mix the raw cacao, oatmeal, 3 tablespoons of the protein powder, peanut butter and 1 tablespoon of chia seed.
2. Form balls
3. Roll in raw cocoa. Put in the fridge 1 hour
4. Serve and enjoy your delicious dessert!

Nutrition facts

Amount per Serving

Calories- 35 g.

Fats- 6.4 g.

Fibre- 3.1 g.

Carbohydrate- 3 g.

Protein- 23 g.

The nutritional details are in general estimate and they should only be used like a guide with approximate use

Recipe 56: Gluten-Free Tiramisu

(Prep time: 8 minutes\ Cook Time: 10 minutes\ Servings: 3)

INGREDIENTS:

For the crumble

- 1 Lightly beaten organic egg
- 1 teaspoon of vanilla extract
- ¼ Cup of melted and cooled coconut oil
- ¼ Cup of coconut sugar
- ½ Cup of coconut flour
- ¼ Cup of almond flour

For the filling:

- 5 Oz of dark chocolate chips + 2 Oz for garnishing
- 1/3 Cup of almond butter
- 3 Tablespoons of coconut cream
- 1 Cup of espresso

DIRECTIONS

1. Start by making the crumble for the tiramisu and to do that make sure you first preheat the oven to about 350° F
2. In a large bowl, mix the beaten egg with the melted and the cooled coconut oil, the coconut sugar and the vanilla extract

3. Add in the almond flour with the coconut flour and mix very well until the form of dough is obtained
4. Spread the dough over a baking sheet lined with a parchment paper and bake for about 12 to 15 minutes
5. Let the baked dough rest for about 10 minutes; then transfer it to a rack until it is cool
6. Break your crust with a fork or with a food processor or simply with a rolling pin
7. Melt the chocolate chips with the almond butter in an oven-safe microwave
8. Stir the chocolate in a mascarpone; then smooth it with a spatula
9. Place a layer of crumbled crumble in the bottom of 4 glasses and sprinkle it with coffee
10. Cover with a layer of chocolate; then with a layer of crumble soaked with coffee
11. Refrigerate for about 3 hours
12. Serve and enjoy your tiramisu!

Nutrition facts
Amount per Serving
Calories- 122.7 g.
Fats- 6.4 g.
Fibre- 3.1 g.
Carbohydrate- 3 g.
Protein- 23 g.

The nutritional details are in general estimate and they should only be used like a guide with approximate use

Recipe 57: Oven Baked Apples

(Prep time: 4 minutes\ Cook Time: 30 minutes\ Servings: 5)

INGREDIENTS

- 5 apples
- 1 Cup of raisins
- ¼ Cup of walnuts
- ¼ Teaspoon of cinnamon
- ½ Teaspoon of natural vanilla extract
- ½ Cup of water

Directions:

1. Heat your oven to about 375° F; then core the apples and pierce it with the help of a fork
2. Mix the raisins, the nuts, cinnamon, and the vanilla in a bowl
3. Fill the centre of the apples with the prepared mixture of the fruits
4. Put the stuffed apples into a glass baking tray; then cover the tray with an aluminium foil paper
5. Bake the apples for around 30 minutes in the oven
6. Serve and enjoy!

Nutrition facts
Amount per Serving
Calories- 119.3 g.

Fats- 4.2 g.
Fibre- 2.1 g.
Carbohydrate- 13 g.
Protein- 2 g.

*The nutritional details are in general estimate and they
should only be used like a guide with approximate use*

Recipe 58: Avocado and Chocolate Mousse

(Prep time: 6 minutes\ Cook Time: 30 minutes\ Servings: 5)

INGREDIENTS

- 2 Peeled; halved and pitted large avocados
- 1/3 Cup of raw honey
- ½ Cup of raw cacao powder
- ¼ Cup of Coconut Milk
- 1/8 Teaspoon of sea salt

Directions:

1. Place your ingredients into a food processor
2. Process your ingredients very well until it becomes smooth
3. Transfer the obtained mixture to a container and refrigerate it for about 1 hour
4. Serve and enjoy your mousse with coconut whipped cream!

Nutrition facts

Amount per Serving

Calories- 253 g.

Fats- 13.3 g.

Fibre- 0.8 g.

Carbohydrate- 12 g.

Protein- 4 g.

The nutritional details are in general estimate and they should only be used like a guide with approximate use

Recipe 59: Chocolate Brownies

(Prep time: 10 minutes\Cook Time: 35 minutes\ Servings: 7-8)

INGREDIENTS

- ½ Cup of almond butter
- ¼ Cup of melted coconut oil
- ¾ Cup of raw organic honey
- ½ of mashed banana
- 1 Tablespoon of vanilla extract
- 1 Cup of Almond Meal/Flour
- ¼ Cup of cacao powder
- 1 Teaspoon of baking soda
- ¼ Teaspoon of salt
- 4 Oz of sugar-free chocolate chips
- 4 Oz of chopped walnuts

Directions:

1. Preheat your oven to a temperature of about 350° F.
2. Grease a baking tray with a little bit of avocado oil
3. Mix altogether the almond butter with the melted coconut oil
4. Add the honey; then egg; the vanilla extract
5. Into another bowl; mix altogether the almond flour; the honey

6. Crack in the egg and the vanilla extract into a small bowl.
7. In another small bowl; mix the almond flour with the cacao powder; the baking soda and the salt
8. Add the dry ingredients to the wet ingredients; then stir very well
9. Add in the chocolate chips and the chopped walnuts
10. Spread your batter evenly into a baking tray; then bake it in the oven at a temperature of about 350° F for about 35 minutes
11. Let your baked tray cool; then cut it into about 16 squares
12. Serve and enjoy your brownies!

Nutrition facts
Amount per Serving
Calories- 205 g.
Fats- 17.5 g.
Fibre- 1 g.
Carbohydrate- 11 g.
Protein- 4.8 g.

The nutritional details are in general estimate and they should only be used like a guide with approximate use

Recipe 60: Zucchini, Chocolate Bread

(Prep time: 5 minutes\cook Time: 35 minutes\ Servings: 7-8)

INGREDIENTS

- 2 Cups of almond meal or almond flour
- 1 Cup of shredded zucchini
- 1 and ½ teaspoons of baking powder
- ¼ Cup of melted coconut oil
- ¼ Cup of ground Chia
- ¾ Cup of water
- ¾ Cup of apple sauce
- 1 Tablespoon of vanilla extract
- 1 Tablespoon of ground cinnamon
- ¼ Cup of maple syrup
- ⅓ Cup of dark chocolate chips

Directions:

1. Preheat your oven to a temperature of about 350° F
2. Grease a medium bread pan
3. Now, substitute an egg by mixing ¼ cup of Chia into a bowl; then mix it very well with ¾ cup of water
4. Now, strain the zucchini and squeeze out any extra quantity of water
5. Mix all together the almond meal, the zucchini, the baking soda, the coconut oil, the

applesauce, the vanilla extract, the cinnamon, the maple syrup, and the Chia egg; then mix with a spatula
6. Fold in the dark chocolate chips; then mix very well
7. Bake your batter in the oven for about 35 to 40 minutes
8. Remove from the oven; then slice the bread
9. Serve and enjoy your bread!

Nutrition facts

Amount per Serving

Calories- 166.2 g.

Fats- 13.18 g.

Fibre- 1.2 g.

Carbohydrate- 5.3 g.

Protein- 8 g.

The nutritional details are in general estimate and they should only be used like a guide with approximate use

CHAPTER 12: CONCLUSION

If you are a beginner to the Ketogenic diet and you have recently adopted it to change your life for the better, this book will make a handy addition to your bookshelf. Not only this book will provide you with everything you need to know about the Ketogenic diet, but it will also offer you a wide variety of recipes that vary from breakfast recipes to lunch recipes, to dinner recipes, snacks, sides, and even desserts.

I have tried to offer you easy-to-make recipes that only need a few and affordable ingredients that can be accessed by everyone alike. And in addition to a large variety of recipes, I have also provided you with the nutrition information of each recipe, so that you won't have to waste so much time in counting the calories, fats, carbohydrates, and fibres.

After reading this cookbook, you will be able to choose which recipes suit you the most, and you will learn what ingredients you should use and what ingredients you should eliminate to maintain a healthy body. It is high time to cut out with all the conventional diets you are used to and learn how to control your carbohydrate intake without calculations. After downloading this book, you will find the best solution to lose weight and prevent the danger of many diseases.

This Ketogenic diet cookbook is extremely easy to use and it will professionally guide you throughout your first experience with the Ketogenic diet. And if you are not new to the Ketogenic diet, then you will find some easy and nice recipes that you will incredibly enjoy.

With 60 Ketogenic recipes, you will figure out that the Ketogenic diet is more than a concept. This comprehensive cookbook will also offer you some tips on using the Ketogenic diet and on what to eat and what to avoid as well.

.

Thanks for Reading our book

I am very glad and proud that I have been able to offer you this book and I hope you have benefited from reading it. If you liked the recipes I have included in this book, please feel free to share it with your friends and family. I value your reviews and I am open to hearing it, and if you have new ideas, don't hesitate to share it with me.
You won't regret reading my recipe book, and don't forget to keep following the upcoming books for a healthier life!